God's diet for
HEALTHY
LIVING

God's diet for
HEALTHY
LIVING

living long, healthy,
and prosperous

AKEAM SIMMONS

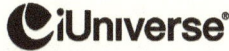

GOD'S DIET FOR HEALTHY LIVING
LIVING LONG, HEALTHY, AND PROSPEROUS

The information, ideas, and suggestions in this book are not intended
as a substitute for professional medical advice. Before following any
suggestions contained in this book, you should consult your personal
physician. Neither the author nor the publisher shall be liable or responsible
for any loss or damage allegedly arising as a consequence of your use
or application of any information or suggestions in this book.

iUniverse books may be ordered through booksellers or by contacting:

iUniverse
1663 Liberty Drive
Bloomington, IN 47403
www.iuniverse.com
1-800-Authors (1-800-288-4677)

ISBN: 978-1-4917-5128-2 (sc)
ISBN: 978-1-4917-5129-9 (e)

Printed in the United States of America.

iUniverse rev. date: 11/14/2014

Scripture quotations marked KJV are from the Holy Bible, King James Version
(Authorized Version). First published in 1611. Quoted from the KJV Classic
Reference Bible, Copyright © 1983 by The Zondervan Corporation.

To Jehovah
The most High God

CONTENTS

God never designed for man to grow old
Man was to live long but not grow old
Old age is a side effect of how you
lived and what you ate
Thus, is the reason why Joshua at 80 still
had the strength of 40, and why many men
in the Old Testament still had children when
they were way over a 100 years old.
Eat right and live right
And you can reduce the side effect-old age
Live long and not grow old!!!!

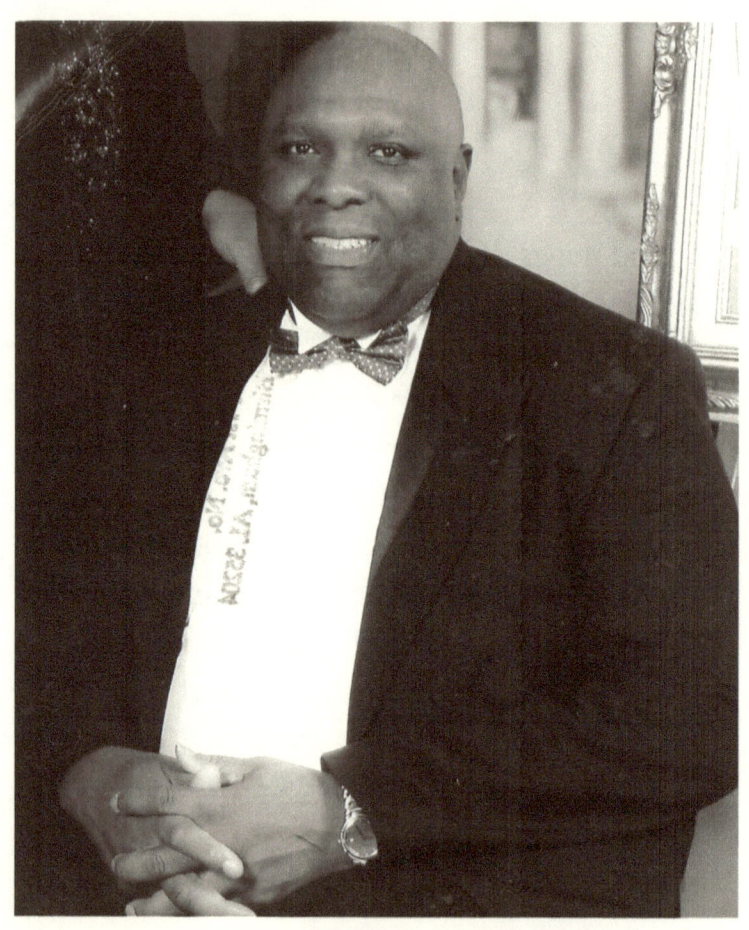

Before weight lost…...295 pounds

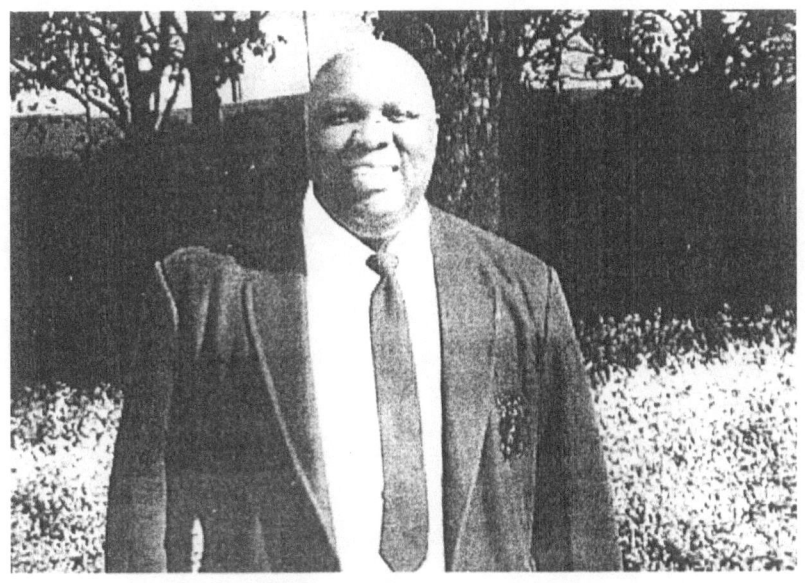

Before weight lost………295 pounds

FOREWORD

There is a problem; an alarming problem that is pervading our streets at an alarming rate, and growing faster than we care to even imagine; a problem that have crossed racial, ethnic, cultural, and national boundaries; causing the whole of us to be effected by it in one way or another. It is the increasing problem of OBESITY. It perhaps is linked to more deaths, particularly in the United States, than any other thing. It ignites heart disease, strokes, depression, cancer, diabetes, and a host of many other death ridden diseases.

The medical world defines obesity as a condition in which excess body fat has accumulated in the body to the extent that it may have an adverse effect on a person's health, which if not addressed adequately, will lead to complications, or even premature death. It is an excess proportion of total body fat. One is considered obese when their weight is 20% or more above suggested weight.

All of our lives, we've been trained to eat wrong, and we've even been told that fat is healthy. When we went home to visit, and Mama saw us at our suggested weight, she would say to us that we needed to put on some weight because we looked puny and unhealthy; so, with that mentality, many Americans dig their graves with their spoons.

It is an inherent problem because usually if mama and daddy are obese, then there is a strong possibility that their children will be overweight and obese also; for we are creatures of happy. We learn by imitating others; thus, we attain bad eating habits from those that are closes to us.

More than 2/3 of adult African Americans are overweight or obese, but, we cannot fully blame Black American for their bad eating habits because it was first forced upon their ancestors as a way to survive. During slavery, the only thing that the slave had to eat was the things that the slave master didn't want and had thrown away. When the slave master slew a hog, cow, or other farm animals, he would leave for the slaves only the parts that he deemed no good- hog intestines, ears, tails, chicken fingers, backs etc. The slaves learned to take those leftovers and live off of them, but they didn't only learn to live on the leftovers, they learned how to make those throw away parts taste good; which is where we get chitterlings (hog's intestines) from.

The problem is, when Black Americans left slavery, they didn't leave the old bad habits; so right now, many blacks still eat chitterlings, fat back, hog malls, and a host of other high in fat foods because they say that they just taste good. Our hospitals and doctors offices are filled with people that are suffering from the effects of too much of these bad for you, but taste good foods; and though these high fat foods were developed from slavery, they are now not just the food choice of the African Americans-for many Caucasians love these foods that are high in fat and calories;

Too, we cannot leave out the other lethal food group besides fatty foods that's killing Americans. It is glucose that is commonly called sugar. Sugar roots began as a rich man's choice-he could afford it. The poor man couldn't afford sugar; the few times that he did taste it, it was a luxury. But, as time past, and sugar become more plenteous, and the United States experienced more wealth, and became one of the most wealthiest nation in the world, hoards of sugar began to invade and penetrate our houses and way of living; thus, too much consumption of sugar gave rise to one of the most lethal diseases of the 20th century-diabetes.

Obesity, because of bad eating habits, is an epidemic in the United States, and what gives rise to this is that we, as Americans, are less active than we were in the past. Modern technology has caused us to be less active and spend less energy. Instead of outside running and bike riding, now, our children, as well as ourselves, are inside sitting down playing some computerized game which usually only gives their fingers a workout. Adults spend their time on the couch watching TV, or on the computer.

Statistics of the Centers for Disease Control and Prevention show that 73% of adults and 43% of children, in the United States, are overweight or obese. And, the statistics are even higher among African Americans-partly because many African Americans view being overweight as a part of their culture. Many black men are attracted to thick black women with large round apple bottom buttocks and thick curvy hips and large breast. Mind you, I am not suggesting African American woman that possess the apple bottom and curvy hips should try to get rid of them, but rather, they should possess the apple bottom and curves with good health; nothing is more attractive than to see a woman with an apple bottom on a small waist, and curves accented by a flat stomach.......my personal opinion, of course!

I might add here, too, that all of us cannot be a size 0, 2, or 6. God didn't design for all of us to be the same size. There are a host of considerations that we must account for when considering our weight; such as height, age, and heredity. One of our biggest problems is that we're often times trying to be the size of somebody else. As stated earlier, God didn't design us to all be one size. You must know you! I am told that at 5'11 I am supposed to weigh around 165 pounds, but I know that 165 is far too small for me; far I am very muscular with broad shoulders and a small waist-a 165 pounds wouldn't look good on me. It is not healthy to try and put a small body on a large frame; so know you, and work towards what's best and comfortable for you.

Usually, when we turn fifty, we don't have the same weight that we had when we were twenty-five. Our metabolism has slowed down, and we're usually not as active at fifty as we were at twenty-five. Thus, we burn fewer calories, but, at the very same time, we eat a little more at fifty than we did at twenty-five, so this means that we are apt to gain weight.

God designed this to be so; for as we age, our body's reproduction of new cells slows down; so we retain some body weight that we didn't usually have because the body is trying to maintain and preserve itself.

Thus, is the reason why Grandma doesn't have the 36-24-36 or the 38-24-42 figure that she use to have, and why Granddaddy doesn't still have that 28 inch waist and sculptured chest that he use to have when he was twenty-five. But, we still can be healthy and look good at any age if we learn to eat right and increase our activity level. Granma might not have the apple bottom buttocks, but she can have a nicely firm buttocks, and still have some wonderful curves if she increase her activities (through exercise), and watch what she eats.

It is our desire, in this book, to attempt to unveil God's design for us in eating and proper living to maintain a good healthy life style. God tells us in the bible what we should eat, and what we should stay away from.

It is our prayer that this book shall be a help to you as you attempt to change your style of life, and become healthier so that you can live a long prosperous life. When you are healthier, not only do you look better, but your body functions better; you think more clearer, and your problem solving abilities increase dramatically.

Chapter One

DIETING

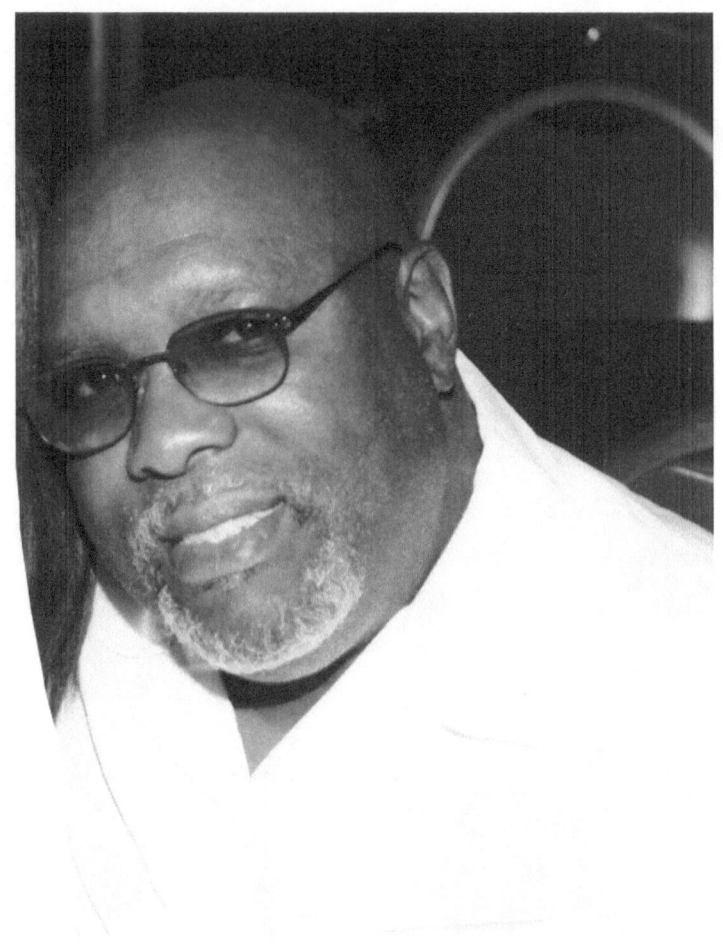

Before weight

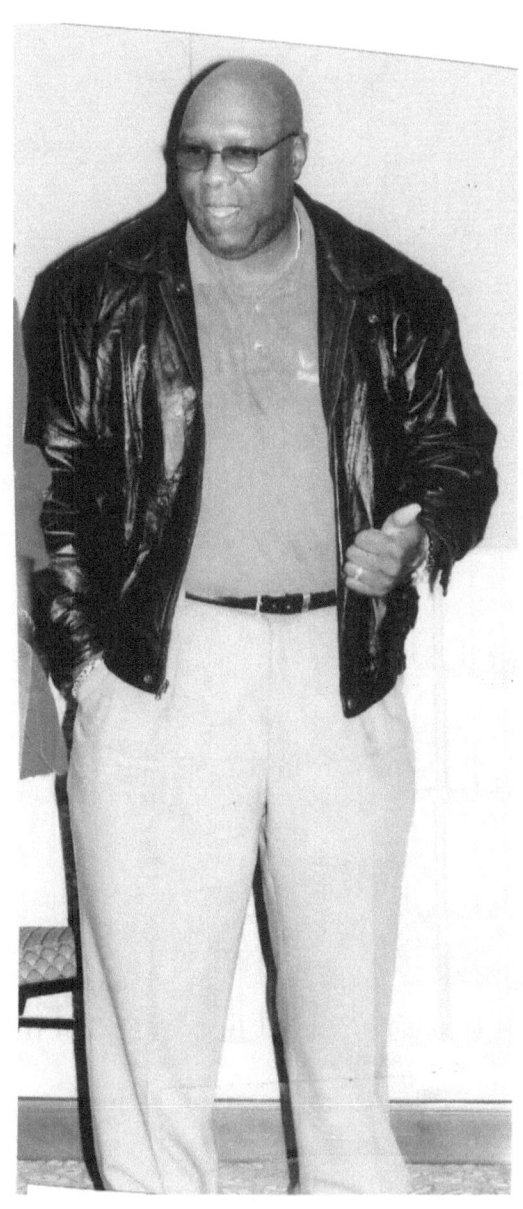

Before weight lost

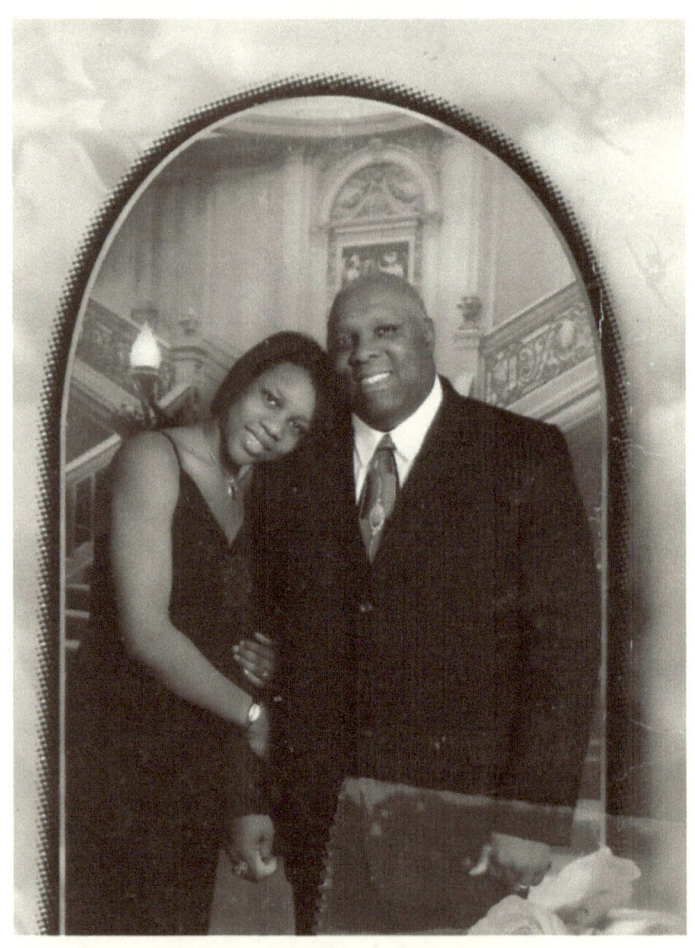

Picture before weight lost

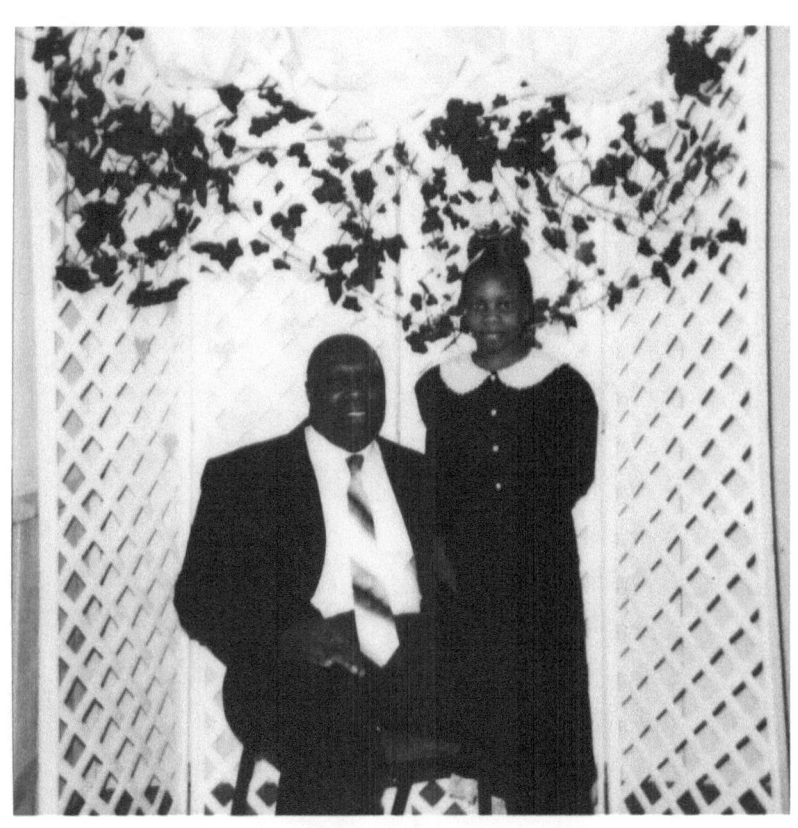

Picture before weight lost

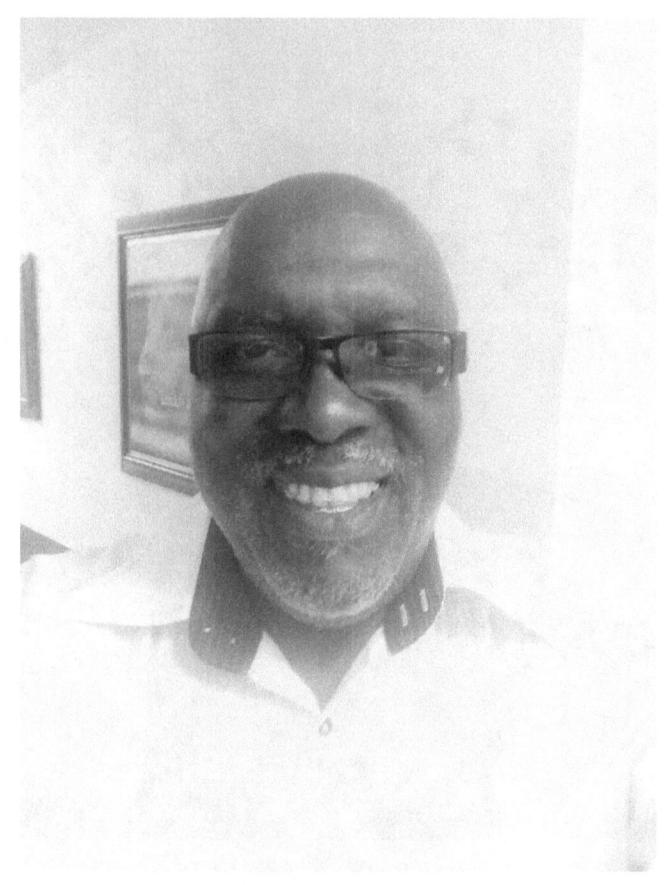

After weight lost

Perhaps, the most wonderful thing about beginning to eat right and losing unwanted pounds is people that are closes to you are affected by your change, and will begin to change too. So, in essence, when you improve your eating habits, you also simultaneously improve the lives of your loved ones. Statistics says that married men live longer; it is partly because married men eat better. Because they have a wife that is usually cooking, or making sure that he eats right, they have a more balanced diet than single men-not to even mention the other bad habits of single men!!

We are often times frightened by the word diet; to some, this word means having to give up all of the good foods that you like to eat, and eat all the foods that nobody likes to eat. But, when you look the word up in the dictionary, the word diet simply means:

1. The usual food and drink of a person or animal.
2. Something eaten or provided regularly

So, thus, your diet is what you eat or drink regularly. All living creature have certain diets; from the lion that eats gazelles, to the elephant that eats shrubbery; from the eagle that eats small game- fish and rodents, to the rabbit that eats vegetables; all are usually eating the same foods regularly, which means that is their diet.

But, to take the word diet a step further, it means:

1. A regulated selection of foods
2. Prescribed food or drink for medical reasons
3. A prescribed food regimen

Number three is the definition that we are mostly focusing on in this book- A prescribed food regimen. A good diet just doesn't happen; it just doesn't fall from the sky; particularly if you are accustomed to having a bad diet. Remember, the two things that stand out most prevalently about us are that we are:

1. Creatures of habit; which simply means that we often times do the same things over and over again-sometimes, even when it is not good for us. For instance, we usually go to the same supermarket; the same gas station; even the same ole way to work every day-because we are creatures of habit; we love familiarity.
2. We are creatures that are prone to immolation. We follow the lead of others. It is in our DNA, right down to our very core. We do what we see others doing. We accept what others find acceptable. We call it our culture, or way of life. Some cultures are offensive to some, but for those who grew up, and accepted it from their forefathers, it is as common as breathing. We

immolate. Statistics show that most educated parents produce educated children; their children don't normally look at higher education as a choice; it is a must! Thus, we often have bad diets because we have been immolating our parents or others close to us.

In order to develop a good diet, we must change our eating habits and change those whose diet we presently immolate.

When I weighed right at 300 pounds, I had a horrible diet, but I thought that I was eating good. Some mornings or afternoons, or whenever I had a taste for some cereal (my favorite was cornflakes), I'd sit down and eat a whole box, or no less than half a box. When I had chicken for dinner, I ate four pieces-that was when I went to the fast food restaurant; I ordered a four piece dinner, but when I ate chicken at home, I'd eat a whole chicken by myself-two legs, two breast, two thighs, two wings, and I'd have sides and deserts with that. A twenty ounce soda was not enough for me, I had to have several with my dinner; if I had tea, the waitress couldn't keep my glass full-I would drink seven or eight glasses of tea. I loved peach cobbler and ice cream. I would eat half of a pie with a quart of ice cream. These are just some of the bad eating habits that I did-all fried food and high sugar intake. I fooled myself that my big frame was muscular, but in essence, I was fat; a huge fat man. When I look at pictures of myself then, I can't believe how I had allowed myself to get so large, and look so bad, but when you look in the mirror, often times, you see what you want to see.

So, DIET, by it self, is not a bad word. Remember, it simply means your eating habits. All living creatures have a diet-whether it's bad or good. They take in substance to maintain living.

When most folks say that their on a diet, they mean that they have chosen a food regimen to help them lose unwanted weight.

Often times, it is no problem doing a chosen diet for a little while, and losing the unwanted poundage, but because we don't make the new diet a way of life, we often times revert back to our old eating habits, and the weight that we had lost, so often comes back; and we usually gain more.

If we properly diet, obesity and overweightness will not be a problem. But, you've got to choose your new good diet, for it does not just happen-and enjoying it won't happen over night. You've got to purposely change your diet, and force yourself to stick to it because in the long run of life, a good diet will help you to live a long, prosperous, and healthy life.

A good diet helps your immune system fight off sickness and disease. You will have fewer sick days if you feed your body the "right" foods-you give your body good weapons to fight sickness and disease (which are your enemies) with. It's like an army; they could go to war with sling shots and sticks and stones-they are weapons, but if your enemies are equipped with guns, then your weapons of choice does little good; so it is with our bodies. We must choose a good diet so that the body will have proper substance to fight foreign intruders (viruses, diseases) with.

When our diet is good, we look younger and more vibrant. Our energy level is more than adequate because we're giving our bodies the right foods through good diet selection; so good cell regeneration is high and functioning adequately.

Choose a good diet, and you choose a better life for you and your loved ones.

PRAY THIS PRAYER FOR STRENGTH:

Father God, great God Jehovah, I thank you for all that you have done in my life and my family life. I even thank you for the times of difficulties, for I know that they were designed to make me stronger. Father, I now ask you to give me the strength that I need over my weaknesses in my flesh; that I'll have strength over my appetite and the foods that I choose in my diet- that they'll be healthy foods that render unto me life and not death. Grant me Godly wisdom in my choice of foods; that I'll be able to enter a healthy weight. In Jesus name I pray-Amen.

Chapter Two

GOD'S DESIGN

**TODAY IS THE BEGINNING
OF THE NEW YOU**

**FIT AND HEALTHY
REAL LASTING CHANGE WILL NOT COME
UNTIL YOU ARE DISSATISFIED WITH YOU
AND UNCOMFORTABLE WHERE YOU ARE**

God didn't just throw man, his creation, together haphazardly. He specifically designed man, and within his design was the diet for man-what he was to eat. From the very first day, God told Adam what was "good" food for him. Notice what God says to Adam about his chosen diet:

Genesis 1: 26-30:

> 26: And God said, let us make man in our image, after our likeness: and let them have dominion over the fish of the sea, and over the fowl of the air, and over the cattle, and over all the earth, and over every creeping thing that creeps upon the earth.

> 27: So God created man in his own image, in the image of God created he him; male and female created he them.

> 28: And God blessed them, and God said unto them, Be fruitful, and multiply, and replenish the earth, and subdue it: and have dominion over the fish of the sea, and over the fowl of the air, and over every living thing that moves upon the earth.

29: And God said, Behold, I have given you every herb bearing seed, which is upon the face of all the earth, and every tree, in the which is the fruit of a tree yielding seed; to you it shall be for meat.

30: And to every beast of the earth, and to every fowl of the air, and to every thing that creeps upon the earth, wherein there is life, I have given every green herb for meat: and it was so.

Note, in the beginning, we were not meat eaters. When he says that herbs and fruit trees were given to man for meat, meat in this sense means food. So, it should read that every herb and fruit tree is given unto you for food.

Animals were also none meat eaters. All of our nourishment was to come from fruits and vegetables; and the animals nourishment was suppose to come from the greeneries of the field.

Originally, we were not designed to be meat eaters!!

When God says that man was suppose to eat herbs and fruit from trees, he was talking about the green plants that have fleshy eatable leaves and stems; that sometimes produce vegetables; the trees bearing fruits, are all fruit trees.

Thus, man's original diet consisted of fruits and vegetables. Then, in the Garden of Eden, he was designed to live forever-never to die; so, we can safely conclude that the original diet that God gave man was a diet designed to give man longevity of life.

Our diet should consist of plenty of fruits and vegetables; as prescribed by our Creator.

Look at how long men lived when they were only eating fruits and vegetables:

Adam (the first man)......930 years old. He had a son, Seth, when he was 130 years old.

Seth (Adam's son)..............912 years old.

Enos.............................905 years old.

Cainan...........................910 years old.

Mahalaleel......................895 years old.

Jared.............................962 years old.

Enoch.........................365 years old.

Enoch didn't die. The bible says that God took him.

Methuselah.....................969 years old.

Methuselah is recorded as living longer than any other man. He was 187 years old when he had his son Lamech.

Lamech..........................777 years old.

Noah.............................950 years old.

Noah didn't have his three sons, Shem, Ham, and Japheth until he was 500 years old.

So, as you can see, seemingly, the body, when its fuel was only fruits and vegetable, it fared better and lived longer. Too, we can safely conclude that their sex drive and other bodily functions were higher. Now –a –days, it is unheard of for a man to have a child at 100 years old, but Noah had three sons after he was 500 years old.

It was not God's design for man to be meat eaters. Man started eating meat after the flood of the earth during Noah's time-after the spiritual fall of man from God. When man fell away from God, he fell out of God's purpose and God's plan; therefore, man was out of God's perfect design for him.

We were never designed to feel the effects of "old age"! Look what the bible records in Deuteronomy 34: 7:

> 7: And Moses was an hundred and twenty years old when he died: his eyes were not dim, nor his natural force abated.

What that is saying is that even though Moses was 120 years old, his eye sight was good, and his body was just as strong as he was when he was younger; in a nut shell, it was saying that Moses did not experience the side effects of old age-in other word, Moses would not have needed eye glasses or bifocals if he lived today.

Caleb was referring to his strength and vitality not diminishing during old age when he spoke to Joshua about his inheritance. Notice what he says, Joshua 14: 6-11:

> 6: Then the children of Judah came unto Joshua in Gilgal: and Caleb the son of Jephunneh the Kenezite said unto him, You know the thing that the Lord said

unto Moses the man of God concerning me and you in Kadesh-barnea.

7: Forty years old was I when Moses the servant of the Lord sent me from Kadesh-barnea to spy out the land; and I brought him word again as it was in my heart.

8: Nevertheless, my brothers that went up with me made the heart of the people melt: but I wholly followed the Lord my God.

9: And Moses swore on that day, saying, Surely the land whereon your feet have trodden shall be your inheritance, and your children's forever; because you have wholly followed the Lord my God.

10: And now, behold, the Lord hath kept me alive, as he said, these forty and five years, even since the Lord spoke this word unto Moses, while the children of Israel wandered in the wilderness: and now, lo, I am this day fourscore and five years old.

11: As yet I am as strong this day, as I was in the day that Moses sent me: as my strength was then, even so is my strength now, for war, both to go out, and to come in.

Caleb is asserting that he was as strong at eighty as he was at forty. He hadn't suffered the side affects of aging.

The bad symptoms that most of us experience during our period of aging are the side affects of a bad diet!

Moses and Joshua were among the last of the children that were transitioning from a fruit and vegetable diet, to a diet that included meat. Thus, is the reason why they didn't live as long as their, fruit and vegetable only, forefathers.

Simply put, it stands to reason that the body does not have to work hard to digest fruits and vegetables. As a matter of fact, some fruits and vegetables contain a great degree of fiber and other digestive molecules to help the body with digesting what it has taken in; and, fruits and vegetables only take a couple of hours to digest.

Meats, on the other hand, take from 12 hours to several days to be digested-some even weeks. So, in essence, that steak that you have Monday can still be with you Tuesday, or even until the next Monday, or even a couple of Mondays (as some suggest). Your body works harder, and expends more energy to digest meats. What adds to digestion time is that your digestive track is about 27 feet long, and your food passes slowly through it- breaking down as it go.

Meats can also introduce you to whatever diseases the animal had. This gives a whole new meaning to the phrase "You are what you eat".

God designed your digestive system to break down, in its smallest terms, any food taken in so it can be adequately used by the body. Your food is broken down into tiny molecular components-usually individual amino acids, simple sugars, and free fatty acids.

Basically, your body has to work much harder to digest meat, particularly beef, because meat is built up mostly of protein-which is harder to break down than other substances.

To reap the best results from our bodies, we must operate it the way that it was designed to function like the Creator made it. We were never made to be meat eaters. Our bodies simply adjusted through the years to tolerate meat, but the consequences have been overly burdensome to your bodies-sickness, disease, and even premature death.

If you can't get rid of meat all together, eat less of it as possible. Adjust to just eating fish and poultry; these are much easier to digest than beef or pork; and if you just got to have some pork or beef, limit yourself. You will live longer and have a better quality of life.

Example, I use to suffer from severe allergies; every week, I'd have an allergy attack. Benadryl became my constant weekly relief. I stopped eating beef and pork for several months, and my allergies stopped completely.

I use to suffer with gout very badly. A couple of times every month, I would have a gout attack-my big toe would swell up, or my entire foot and ankle would swell and become tender to even touch; but after I changed my diet-no beef or pork, and cut down on sugars, and ate plenty of fruits and vegetables, my gout episodes desisted completely.

I can only imagine what other positive effects changing my diet has produce in my body.

God's design for you is to live a productive life. Look what Jesus said in part of John 10: 10:

> 10: I am come that you might have life, and that you might have it more abundantly.

We're not supposed to just survive; we're supposed to have abundant life. This starts with your diet and walking in God's design. It matters little what you shall come to possess if you cannot enjoy it because your body is sick.

Look at God's design in Jeremiah. God said that he has plans for you. Jeremiah 29: 11-12:

> 11: For I know the thoughts that I think towards you, says the Lord, thoughts of peace, and not of evil, to give you an expected end.

> 12: Then shall you call upon me, and you shall go and pray unto me, and I will listen unto you.

God has already designed for us a successful life with a wonderful end. But, he also gives us a choice to choose to live contrary to his purpose. Even though we are saved, and on our way to heaven, we can still live quiet lives of defeat on earth-if we choose to.

He gave us an owner's manual on how to live a successful life and have great success, and even how to eat and live healthy fulfilling lives. Note Ezekiel 4: 9-11:

> 9: Take you also unto you wheat, and barley, and beans, and lentils, and millet, and fitches, and put them in one vessel, and make you bread thereof, according to the number of the days that you shall lie upon your bed, three hundred and ninety days shall you eat thereof.

> 10: And your meat which you shall eat shall be by weight, twenty shekels a day: from time to time shall you eat it.

> 11: You shall drink also water by measure, the sixth part of an hin: from time to time shall you drink.

God was telling his people how to eat during times of troubles and trials to survive. I believe that this kind of eating helps de-stress the body and gives it more energy to operate.

Remember, God's original design for us was to live forever without pain, suffering, sickness, and death. We brought all of these conditions on ourselves. Most of our sickness and disease has to do with our diet (that which we constantly eat); so, change the man's diet, and you change the health of the man.

Live long, healthy, and prosperous is God's design for man-His most wondrous creation; to do that, we must follow God's design, and God's plan. We must look very closely at the diet of early man-when he was living 800 and 900 years. What he ate and how he lived, will give us a clue on how we should eat and how we should live if we too want to live a very long and healthy life.

The Bible says that Moses did not have any of the side affects of growing old. Look what it says: Deuteronomy 34: 5-7:

> 5, So Moses the servant of the Lord died there in the land of Moab, according to the word of the Lord.

> 6. And he buried him in a valley in the land of Moab, over against Beth-pe'-or: but no man knows of his sepulcher unto this day.

7. And Moses was an hundred and twenty
years old when he died: his eyes were not
dim, nor his natural forces abated.

Allow me to make it simple of what that text is saying about Moses and his health. Moses was a 120 years old when he died (what we call an old man), but note what it stresses, his eyes were not dim; which meant that he had perfect vision. He didn't need the assistance of glasses, or any thing to help him see. His vision remained as a young man; then it says that his natural forces were not abated. It means that, Moses, the natural man, natural body did not experience the natural changes that usually accompany a 120 years old man. If this was the norm, then it would have not been worth mentioning. The "natural forces" meant that everything that Moses body could do as a young man, he could also do it as a 120 years old man- Moses didn't suffer from high blood pressure, heart disease, shortness of breath, or even such common things that now plague older men-like certain parts of their bodies stop working, or does not work as well as they did when he was a young man. No, Moses had none of those things that natural men were accustomed to having! I believe that it was mainly because of his Diet and his Relationship with God.

As we have already said, as worth stressing again, note again carefully.

I believe Caleb experienced the same supreme natural forces as Moses did, for look what Caleb says in his conversation to Joshua when asking for an entire mountain for himself. Joshua 14: 9-11:

> 9. And Moses swore on that day, saying, Surely the land whereon your feet have trodden shall be your inheritance, and your children's for ever, because you have wholly followed the Lord my God.

> 10. And now, behold, the Lord has kept me alive, as he said, these forty and five years, even since the Lord spoke this word unto Moses, while the children of Israel wandered in the wilderness: and now, lo, I am this day fourscore and five years old.

> 11. As yet I am as strong this day as I was in the day that Moses sent me: as my strength was then, even so is my strength now, for war, both to go out, and to come in.

Caleb was saying the same thing as is written of Moses-his natural forces had not abated. He was just as strong at 85 years old as he was at 45 years old. He says unto Joshua that he was able to fight just as strongly at 85 years old as he did at 45 years old; and I suspect that if we could research it, he was physically just like Moses-his vision was perfect, and his natural forces never ceased or decreased. Their diet and relationship to God made the difference.

We stressed Mosses and Caleb over and over again to impress upon you the very possibility of living a long life without being plagued by the issues of old age.

What we eat and how we live determines how long we shall live, and what quality of life we shall have. Being 85 and suffering from all kinds of ailments to where one is confined to a bed and needing someone else to take care of you, and your greatest daily conversation is of the ailments of which you suffer, you have little life, and are not LIVING the life that you were designed to live.

God's design for us is to live a long happy, healthy, wealthy life that is full of joy; but to live in God's design, we must change our diets and develop a relationship with our Creator.

PRAY THIS PRAYER FOR STRENGTH:

Oh God, I thank you for giving me the strength to adhere to a healthy diet; now I ask you for strength to walk in what you have designed just for me, for my life. Give me the strength to live in your perfect Will and design for my life. Give me the strength and the vision to see your plan and your design for my life, and the strength and fortitude to walk there in- In Jesus name-Amen.

Chapter Three

DIET TO LIVE

Keep in mind that "diet" is whatever one consistently consume into their body (food or drink). Our diets are what sustains us and gives us the degree of life that we have; thus is the reason why some live long lives with ailments, and others live long lives with few or no ailments; still yet others live short lives filled with sickness and ailments. In either case, most have to do with the individual's diets.

I have personally experienced the healthy benefits of a good diet. A few years ago, I ate anything; pork, beef, lots of fat, lots of sugar, and anything that I felt I had a desire to eat. I weighed a whopping 295 pounds on a 5' 10" frame. I suffered from gout; a few times every month my big toe, foot, or ankle would swell with excruciating pain. I had high blood pressure, high cholesterol, type two diabetes, and severe allergies. I could tell when it was going to rain, for my allergies would always worsen just before the rain. I would sneeze and sneeze and sneeze; my head ached, my eyes ran, my nose was severely stopped up, and I found it difficult to breathe; and when I slept, I snored so loudly until no one close to me could sleep-I sounded like a freight train roaring in the bed room; then, I stumbled upon God's diet for man-His creation. I got on God's diet, and in three months, my allergies were gone; in six months I had no more gout flare ups, and in a year, my high flood pressure and high cholesterol was gone. In two years, on God's diet, I went from weighing 295 pounds to weighing 210 pounds. Did I mess up sometimes along the way, yes, of course, but when I messed up, I got right back on God's diet until it became a way of life for me. Living on the diet that God designed for me, helps to give me a long wealthy and prosperous life that produces wealth, for a healthy body produces a healthy mind, and a healthy mind can always acquire wealth. Health and wealth goes together; for it is misery to have wealth and bad health.

Note the first time that God mentions man and the animals that he had created and his designed diet for them. Genesis 1: 26-30:

> 26. And God said, Let us make man in our image, after our likeness: and let them have dominion over the fish of the sea, and over the fowl of the air, and over the cattle, and over all the earth, and over every creeping thing that creeps upon the earth.

> 27. So God created man in his own image, in the image of God created he them.

> 28. And God blessed them, and God said unto them, Be fruitful, and multiply, and

replenish the earth, and subdue it: and have dominion over the fish of the sea, and over the fowl of the air, and over every living thing that moves upon the earth.

29. And God said, Behold, I have given you every herb bearing seed, which is upon the face of all the earth, and every tree, in the which is the fruit of a tree yielding seed; to you it shall be for meat.

30. And to every beast of the earth, and to every fowl of the air, and to every thing that creeps upon the earth, wherein there is life, I have given every green herb for meat: and it was so.

Note, our original diet only consisted of fruits, vegetables, and herbs. What exactly is an herb? Herbs are any plants used for flavoring, food, medicine. Culinary use typically distinguishes herbs as referring to the leafy green parts of a plant and other parts of the same plant; such as seeds, berries, bark, roots and some fruits.

Herbs also have a medicinal effect upon man when he eats them. It is like eating food and medicine all at the same time. Some herbs, to name of few, are: aloe vera, asparagus, artichoke, basil, bee balm, oregano, ginseng, and hundreds of others. Remember, herbs are usually used to give flavor to other foods, but many can be eaten by themselves.

So, man's original diet was fruits, vegetables, and herbs (not green herbs, for green herbs were for the animals). This is the first diet that God gave to man; the diet that he was given when he was to live forever in the Garden of Eden. God specifically designed man's diet-a diet that would preserve him. Observe the care that God gave the plants and the herbs of the earth for man Genesis 2: 5-9:

> 5: And every plant of the field before it was in the earth, and every herb of the field before it grew: for the Lord God had not caused it to rain upon the earth, and there was not a man to till the ground.

> 6. But there went up a mist from the earth, and watered the whole face of the ground.

> 7. And the Lord God formed man of the dust of the ground, and breathed into

his nostrils the breath of life; and man
became a living soul.

8. And the Lord God planted a garden
eastward in Eden; and there he put the
man whom he had formed.

9. And out of the ground made the Lord
God to grow every tree that is pleasant to
the sight, and good for food; the tree of
life also in the midst of the garden, and
the tree of knowledge of good and evil.

See what care God took of the man that he had made;
how he personally formed the plants and the herbs,
and took specific care of them, for it was never God's
intention for His creation to die.

Man's food supply was everything that grew upon the
trees, or plants, and herbs. Note Genesis 2: 16:

16. And the Lord God commanded the
man, saying, Of every tree of the garden
you may freely eat:

This diet would keep away disease, sickness, and all
kinds of uncomfortable ailments like the ones that
plague man today. The medicines that would keep man

well and prevent any attacks from unwanted viruses, micro organisms, and uninvited inside growths was encapsulated in what he fed himself daily-the daily provisions that God had made-fruits, plants, herbs, and a relationship with him.

Man was never suppose to know what a head ache felt like, or what sickness was, or what cancer, or bodily ailments were; he was not even to ever know what a common cold was. His diet and relationship was a holy designed preventive prescription for wholeness and wellness.

Just imagine a world without a hospital, drug store, undertaker, or cemetery-nobody was suppose to get sick, or die; but then, man, God's creation went contrary to God's instructions. Man straying from God's designed diet is what changed his entire life, and the life of all of mankind that was to come after Adam-the first man.

I submit to you today that just like Adam, what we put in our mouths causes us much harm and duress; as it has often times been said, "We dig our graves with our forks and spoons."

Genesis chapters one and two deals with man's first diet-his diet designed for him to live forever without sickness and disease. His second diet starts in chapter three where God introduces His man to a new diet, and the introduction to bread (As some theologians suppose, I don't believe this introduction of bread simply speaks of man's daily intake of food; no, I believe that it is literally man's first introduction to "Bread"-baked dough from some kind of grain taken from the earth).

Look what God says to Adam when he gives Adam his curse for eating the forbidden food. Genesis 3: 17-19:

> 17. And unto Adam he said, because you have listened unto the voice of your wife, and have eaten of the tree, of which I commanded you, saying, You shall not eat of it: cursed is the ground for your sake; in sorrow shall you eat of it all the days of your life;

> 18. Thorns also and thistles shall it bring forth to you; and you shall eat the herb of the field;

> 19. In the sweat of your face shall you eat bread, till you return unto the ground; for out of it were you taken: for dust you are, and unto dust shall you return.

The second phase of Man's diet was fruits, vegetables, herbs, and bread, but, mind you, bread was not in the original diet. It came after the curse (that's why bread is not good for man-it ushers him towards death; it's a symbol of the curse).

So, before we journey any further in this book, the first phase of our new diet to live is to delete bread from our diets; as long as we're consuming bread, it is facilitating the curse of death upon us!

During this second phase of Adam's diet (the first man), during this curse, Adam still had a son after he was 130 years old, and after he had his son he live 800 years. Thus, Adam's diet afforded him to live 930 years.

The second phase of the first man's diet produced long life among its recipients. It was during this time that the oldest man that ever lived, Methuselah, lived-969 years old. If you read the book of Genesis during that era, it was quite common for people to live to be over 800 and over 900 years old. Even though, during this time, these people lived under the curse, they still had a close relationship with God; for that reason, many of them were still quite healthy, and had their first child after they were well over a hundred years old; some were recorded to have children after they were 500 years old: this is unheard of during our times. In our times, a woman is considered done having children after she turns 40, and no later than 45. As you can see, that diet kept their bodies in a youthful state.

The third phase of man's diet to live came about after the flood. I think that this diet came about more of necessity than of structured design, for it was after the flood of all the earth during Noah's time. Everything, every plant and every tree was dead, thus fruits, vegetables, and the like, were dead and had to be re-grown, which would take many years; so during this third phase, man's diet was altered severely. He was now about to eat that which he had never eaten before-MEAT. The first eating of meat was introduced to man and the animals that survived the flood, for here-to-fore, all ate fruit, vegetable, herbs, and bread of course for the man. Note Genesis 9: 1-4:

> 1. And God blessed Noah and his sons, and said unto them, Be fruitful, and multiply, and replenish the earth.

> 2. And the fear of you and the dread of you shall be upon every beast of the earth, and upon every fowl of the air, upon all that moves upon the earth, and upon all

the fishes of the sea; into your hand are they delivered.

3. Every moving thing that lives shall be meat for you; even as the green herb have I given you all things.

4. But flesh with the life thereof, which is the blood thereof, shall you not eat.

During this third diet phase, man ceased being a vegetarian, and became a meat eater, but even becoming a meat eater there were stipulations given him-mainly that he could not eat anything raw, or eat anything that was still alive; that also means that his meat should not be rare-for rare is raw, and sometimes still has the blood running from it upon your plate.

All of God's diets were for man's benefit. The first diet was design for him to live forever in the Garden of Eden, under the hand of God where he could walk with God and physically see God. In Eden, he could bath in God's glory every day, and he could speak to God face to face.

You see, Adam was not the first man that God had placed upon the earth-he was the next man that God had created to dwell upon the earth. God had destroyed the man before Adam. I can safely come to this conclusion because of what God first says to Adam, and what he first says to Noah after the flood. Note the two. Genesis 1: 28:

> 28. And God blessed them, and God said unto them, Be fruitful, and multiply, and replenish the earth, and subdue it: and have dominion over the fish of the sea, and over the fowl of the air, and over every living thing that moves upon the earth.

Genesis 9: 1:

> 1. And God blessed Noah and his sons, and said unto them Be fruitful, and multiply, and replenish the earth.

He tells both of them to REPLENISH. Now to replenish, means that something, or some bodies had to have been before and was taken off the seen for whatever reason. You cannot redo something that had not already been done; so he tells Adam and Noah to replenish after everything had been destroyed.

The third diet was afforded Noah so that he could live and replenish the earth; remember, the only thing that he had in abundance was meat-the animals on the ship with him, but note, in the third diet, God tells man to eat green herbs. During the first and second phases of man's diets, man was not given green herbs to eat. It was only for the animals. Here, He instructs him to add green herb to his diet. Why? I submit to you that it was for medicinal reasons.

Diet one, we were to live forever in the presence of God. Diet two, we were extracted from his presence and bread was added to our diets (the cursed thing); and at the start of the third diet, we are introduced to a new diet-meat and green herbs. Man did not need the medicinal powers of the green herb prior to the flood of Noah's time because he lived in the presence of God; so enjoyed the benefits of God's healing hand upon his life-and he only ate fruits, vegetables, herbs, and bread.

The third diet comes because he is introduced to eating something that would be hard on his body and cause his digestive system to change drastically-for now, it had to breakdown meat so the body could use it as fuel. The green herb was for the curing or halting the side effects of man's consumption of meat. Thus, if you eat meats, you must also have a diet rich in herbs and green herbs. Season your meat with green herbs; for there lies the disease fighters that fight cancer, tumors, blood diseases, and all manner of ailments that comes from digesting meat.

Observe too, that God tells man at that time that he was allowed to eat every moving thing that lives upon the earth; that meant that man had no restrictions on what he could eat. If he could catch it, he could eat it-whatever animal that lived-snakes, birds, bugs, fish, hogs, pigs, cows, horses, insects, etc. All things living and moving was upon man's diet; but it had to be consumed amidst green herbs.

This principle is still alive today! If you eat any sort of meats, it has to be accompanied by green herbs and spices; herbs like: flax seed, oregano, basil, ginseng, cinnamon, cardamom, cloves, dill weed, pepper, parsley, etc.

For every sickness and disease that man has, or will have, there is a herb or spice that can cure it; the problem is finding the right herb or spice.

Remember, I had gout, high blood pressure, type two diabetes, and severe allergies, but when I changed my diet, and filled it with plenty of herbs and spices, all of those ailments went away. I might add here too that I had had a severe herniated disc in my neck. If I turned my neck too fast, the disc would pop out and cause my neck to immediately become stiff, where I could not turn my head without turning my shoulders; I could sneeze, and the herniated disc would pop out. The doctor told me that there was no fix for the herniated disc in my neck outside of surgery; but when I changed my diet, and stopped eating meat, consumed lots of vegetables, and added plenty of herbs and spices to my diet, my herniated disc simply went away.

Having looked at the benefits of herbs and spices, it is no wonder that the early men of the earth lived exceptionally long lives. They had a diet full of fruits and vegetables, and rich with herbs and spices.

If we are to get the fullness of our lives, and live long, healthy, and prosperous lives, we have got to immolate our early forefathers, and eat lots of vegetables and fruits; if we eat meat, it has to be seasoned with herbs and spices (our vegetables too). But, **the lesser the meat in your diet, the better your body functions!!!!!**

PRAY THIS PRAYER FOR STRENGTH:

Lord grant me the strength to resist those foods for which I found pleasure in; those foods that I was taught to eat; give me the strength to select lots of fruits and vegetables, and limit my intake of meats-particularly those meats that are detrimental to my health. Let me evolve into enjoying those foods that are good for me, and let me acquire a taste for them. I claim strength over my weakness right now. I am strong with the strength that God has given me-in Jesus name-Amen.

Chapter Four

THE FOURTH DIET

Previously, after man had come out of the flood, and most of the plant life was dead, God, in His third diet, allowed man to eat anything that moved on the earth; then, in the book of Deuteronomy, after everything had been revived, He starts His fourth diet which he meticulously lays out for man-which animals he can eat and which animals he cannot. Observe Deuteronomy 14: 3-21:

3. You shall not eat any abominable thing.

4. These are the beasts which you shall eat: the ox, the sheep, and the goat,

5. The hart, and the roebuck, and the fallow deer, and the wild goat, and the pygarg, and the wild ox, and the chamois.

6. And every beast that parts the hoof, and leaves the cleft into two claws, and chews the cud among the beasts, that you shall eat.

7. Nevertheless these you shall not eat of them that chew the cud, or of them that divide the cloven hoof; as the camel, and the hare, and the coney; for they chew

the cud, but divide not the hoof; therefore they are unclean unto you.

8. And the swine, because it divides the hoof, yet chews not the cud, it is unclean unto you: you shall not eat their flesh, nor touch their dead carcass.

9. These you shall eat of all that are in the waters: all that have fins and scales shall you eat:

10. And whatsoever have not fins and scales you may not eat; it is unclean unto you.

11. Of all clean birds you shall eat.

12. But these are they of which you shall not eat: the eagle, and the ossifrage, and the ospray,

13. And the glede, and the kite, and the vulture after his kind,

14. And every raven after his kind,

15. And the owl, and the night hawk, and the cuckow, and the hawk after his kind,

16. The little owl, and the great owl, and the swan.

17. And the pelican, and the gier eagle, and the cormorant,

18. And the stork, and the heron after her kind, and the lapwing, and the bat.

19. And every creeping thing that flies is unclean unto you; they shall not be eaten.

20. But of all clean fowls you may eat.

21. You shall not eat of any thing that dies of itself; you shall give it unto the stranger that is in your gates, that he may eat it; or you may sell it unto an alien: for you are an holy people unto the Lord your God. You shall not seethe a kid in his mother's milk.

This forth diet actually starts in the book of Leviticus; Deuteronomy mirrors it, and it perhaps includes a little more information upon the animals of which we can eat, or not eat. Note what it says. Leviticus 11: 2-47:

> 2. Speak unto the children of Israel, saying, These are the beasts which you shall eat among all the beasts that are on the earth.

> 3. Whatsoever parts the hoof, and is cloven foot, and chews the cud, among the beasts, that shall you eat.

> 4. Nevertheless these shall you not eat of them that chew the cud, or of them that divide the hoof: as the camel, because he chews the cud, but divides not the hoof; he is unclean unto you.

> 5. And the coney, because he chews he cud, but divides not the hoof; he is unclean unto you.

> 6. And the hare, because he chews the cud, but divides not hoof; he is unclean unto you.

7. And the swine, though he divide the hoof, and be cloven foot, yet he chews not the cud; he is unclean to you.

8. Of their flesh shall you not eat, and their carcass shall you not touch; they are unclean to you.

9. These shall you eat of all that are in the waters: Whatsoever have fins and scales in the waters, in the seas, and in the rivers, them shall you eat.

10. And all that have not fins and scales in the seas, and in the rivers, of all that move in the waters, and of any living thing which is in the waters, they shall be an abominations unto you:

11. They shall be even an abomination unto you; you shall not eat of their flesh, but you shall have their carcass in abomination.

12. Whatsoever has no fins nor scales in the waters, that shall be an abomination unto you.

13. And these are they which you shall have in abomination among the fowls; they shall not be eaten, they are an abomination: the eagle, and the ossifrage, and the ospray,

14. And the vulture, and the kite after his kind;

15. Every raven after his kind;

16. And the owl, and the night hawk, and the cuckow, and the hawk after his kind,

17. And the little owl, and the cormorant, and the great owl,

18. And the swan, and the pelican, and the gier eagle,

19. And the stork, the heron after her kind, and the lapwing, and the bat.

20. All fowls that creep, going upon all four, shall be an abomination unto you.

21. Yet these may you eat of every flying creeping thing that goes upon all four,

which have legs above the feet, to leap with upon the earth;

22. Even these of them you may eat; the locust after his kind, and the bald locust after his kind, and the beetle after his kind, and the grasshopper after his kind.

23. But all other flying creeping things, which have four feet, shall be an abomination unto you.

24. And for these you shall be unclean: whosoever touches the carcass of them shall be unclean until the even.

25. And whosoever bears ought of the carcass of them shall wash his clothes, and be unclean until the even.

26. The carcass of every beast which divides the hoof, and is not cloven foot, nor chews the cud, are unclean unto you: every one that touches them shall be unclean.

27. And whatsoever goes upon his paws, among all manner of beasts that go on all

four, those are unclean unto you: whoso touches their carcass shall be unclean until the even.

28. And he that bears the carcass of them shall wash his cloths, and be unclean until the even: they are unclean unto you.

29. These also shall be unclean unto you among the creeping things that creep upon the earth; the weasel, and the mouse, and the tortoise after his kind,

30. And the ferret, and the chameleon, and the lizard, and the snail, and the mole.

31. These are unclean to you among all that creep: whosoever does touch them, when they be dead, shall be unclean until the even.

32. And upon whatsoever any of them, when they are dead, does fall, it shall be unclean; whether it be any vessel of wood, or raiment, or skin, or sack, whatsoever vessel it be, wherein any work is done, it must be put into water, and it shall

be unclean until the even; so it shall be cleansed.

33. And every earthen vessel, where into any of them falls, whatsoever is in it shall be unclean; and ye shall break it.

34. Of all meat which may be eaten, that on which such water comes shall be unclean: and all drink that may be drunk in every such vessel shall be unclean.

35. And every thing where upon any part of their carcass falls shall be unclean; whether it be oven, or ranges for pots, they shall be broken down: for they are unclean, and shall be unclean unto you.

36. Nevertheless a fountain or pit, wherein there is plenty of water, shall be clean: but that which touches their carcass shall be unclean.

37. And if any part of their carcass fall upon any sowing seed which is to be sown, it shall be clean.

38. But if any water be put upon the seed, and any part of their carcass fall thereon, it shall be unclean unto you.

39. And if any beast, of which you may eat, die; he that touches the carcass thereof shall be unclean until the even.

40. And he that eats of the carcass of it shall wash his clothes, and be unclean until the even: he also that bears the carcass of it shall wash his clothes, and be unclean until the even.

41. And every creeping thing that creeps upon the earth shall be an abomination; it shall not be eaten.

42. Whatsoever goes upon the belly, and whatsoever goes upon all four, or whatsoever has more feet among all creeping things that creeps upon the earth, them you shall not eat, for they are an abomination.

43. You shall not make your selves abominable with any creeping thin that creeps, neither shall you make yourselves

unclean with them, that you should be defiled thereby.

44. For I am the Lord your God: you shall therefore sanctify yourselves, and you shall be holy; for I am holy: neither shall you defile yourselves with any manner of creeping thing that creeps upon the earth.

45. For I am the Lord that brings you up out of the land of Egypt, to be your God: you shall therefore be holy, for I am holy.

46. This is the law of the beasts, and of the fowl, and of every living creature that moves in the waters and of every creature that creeps upon the earth:

47. To make a difference between the unclean and the clean, and between the beast that may be eaten and the beast that may not be eaten.

God is quite more meticulous about man's diet in Leviticus than he is in Deuteronomy. He often times refers to different foods that are an abomination to man, which simply means that whichever food is abominable it does not agree with you, more importantly, it attracts other unwanted things to you. In other words, any food that God refers to as an abomination is not good for you and it causes diseases, sickness, and ailments. It is the reason why we have pervasive cancer everywhere, tumors growing in the body in places they shouldn't, and the body's immune system fail and breakdown.

When you eat something that's abominable, it tares down your body's natural defenses, and invite other harmful micros into your body which fights healthy cells; so pay very particular attention to the foods that God says is an abomination to you. It is not that God simply does not like the food; it is God warning you that it is not good for you, and that because of those foods, you will have unwanted sickness and diseases.

Staying away from abominable foods pleases God, and puts us in a position of favor with God. Observe what the prophet Ezekiel says about this in the book of Ezekiel 4: 14:

> 14. Then said I, Ah Lord God! Behold, my soul has not been polluted: for from my youth up even till now have I not eaten of that which dies of itself, or is torn in pieces; neither came there abominable flesh into my mouth.

Ezekiel's stance was he had observed his diet, and hadn't eaten anything that was abominable or defiled (defiled means unfit), or unclean-unclean simply refers to that which contaminates your body.

When we eat all of these foods that God has told us is not good for us, then we pollute our bodies-like a polluted river, it has all kinds of unnatural stuff floating in it-stuff that often times carry germs and bacteria.

Although God's eating design for us has a spiritual connotation, it just naturally makes sense, for you consume whatever the animal you are eating has consumed; so thus it makes sense that God would tell us that the only fish that we are to eat has to have fins and scales-every thing else is not good for us.

Think about it. Shrimp, lobster, crab, squid, scallops, cat fish, dolphin, shark, whale, oysters, claims, etc, all is not good for our bodies. They invite other microbes that carry disease to come into us and set up house. I suspect that one of the reasons why they are not good for us is that basically they are scavengers-they eat whatever they find, dead or alive; and many of them scavenge upon the bottom of the sea, eating whatever the other animals waist and excrete from their bodies.

Note too, God says that even handling the defiled and abominable creatures will make you unclean (expose you to things that are not good for you); so He tells us that when we handle such creatures, go and wash yourselves thoroughly.

Remember it was and still is God's design for us to prosper and be in good health, but he never takes away our ability to choose what we want-even when it is not good for us.

You have got to make the choice right now today to push aside all those unclean, defile, and abominable foods from you that are reeking sickness and death in your life.

PRAY THIS PRAYER FOR STRENGTH:

Father God, I thank you for teaching me the foods that are good for me and those that are not; I thank you for showing me what to eat to live a long and healthy life. Thank you for giving me the strength to pull off all of those old bad eating habits that I was taught. I choose to stay away from the unclean beast and the defiled animals that ushers me towards death and sickness. I choose this day to live without the sicknesses that eating defiled and unclean animals bring. I choose life over death-In Jesus name-Amen.

Chapter Five

ABIDING BY THE LAW

When we break the law, whether natural or spiritual, there are dire consequences. To the degree that we break the law is the equal degree of consequences that we suffer. In the natural law, you wouldn't be given twenty years in prison for running a stop sign, nor would one just be given a ticket if one had murdered someone. The consequences equal the offence.

If you blatantly disregard the laws, you pay severely!

God has set up laws that we should abide by, and when we fail to, we pay the price. Like, for example, the law of gravity. It does not matter who you are, if you break this law, you pay to the degree that you broke it. The law of gravity is designed to keep things upon the earth so that they don't just float off into space. If there was no law of gravity, with gravitational pull, then everything that wasn't nailed down would just float away.

When we step up on a box or latter, and jump off, we just broke the law of gravity, so the law of gravity pulls us out of the air and onto the ground. The consequences of breaking the gravity law by jumping off of the box is gravity pulls us down to the earth, but the consequences are so little until we feel little or no effect from the sudden hit to the ground. If you were to ascend to a twenty story building and jump, breaking the law of gravity, then the law of gravity will immediately pull you down to the earth at an alarming speed. You would die from the impact of hitting the earth and stopping so suddenly-it is the price you pay for breaking the law of gravity to that degree.

We also have laws that govern our society, and when one breaks the laws of society, then society forces one to pay a price. If the law says that you can only drive 35 miles an hour in a certain area, and you go and drive above that, then you are breaking the driving law and subject to a fine.

If one throws paper onto the side of the road, then one is breaking the litter law, and is subject to penalty for breaking the law.

Law simply means that which regulates the actions and administer consequences.

God says that there is a food law; it regulates our eating habits. If we abide by the law, we live a long healthy life, but if we break the law, then the consequences are sickness, disease, and all kinds of ailments. When we break the food law, we introduce our bodies to all sorts of micros that attack our cells, and even set up house inside of us-living and killing us slowly daily.

Closely observe what God says about the food law. Leviticus 11: 46-47:

> 46. This is the law of the beasts, and of the fowl, and of every living creature that moves in the waters, and of every creature that creeps upon the earth:

> 47. To make a difference between the unclean and the clean, and between the beast that may be eaten and the beast that may not be eaten.

If we abide by God's food law, we live healthy and long. The things that we connect with old age are simply the side effects of breaking God's eating law. Wrinkled skin, bad vision, arthritis, memory lost, bending over, weakness, moving slowly, shortness of breath, aches and pains, etc, are all things that we assume is a part of growing old, but when we take a closer look, they are, in fact, the side effects of breaking God's eating law. Most folks are, in essence, slowly committing suicide every day.

If we didn't break God's eating law, there would be no such thing as "old folk"; there would simply be people that live a long time, and you couldn't look at them and tell their ages; and when they died, they would just sleep away-as Moses did.

Many confuse scripture, and think that they have been given allowance to eat anything as long as they pray over it and bless it before they put it in their months; but this action is a misunderstanding and a misinterpretation of scripture.

Look at what Jesus says in Mark 16: 17-18:

> 17. And these signs shall follow them that believe; In my name shall they cast out devils; they shall speak with new tongues;

> 18. They shall take up serpents; and if they drink any deadly thing, it shall not hurt them; they shall lay hands on the sick, and they shall recover.

Now pay particular attention to where Jesus says that if they drink any deadly thing, it shall not hurt them. If we take this literally as is, we would come up with the understanding that we can drink poison, and it won't hurt us, but after careful examination of this text, he is not saying that at all. He is saying that during their quest to serve Him, amidst their ministry, if they should "unknowingly" drink poison or any deadly liquid, it shall not hurt them.

If they knowingly drink a deadly thing, it will kill them! Jesus was promising them protection during ministry, not an allowance to simply break God's eating law.

Another place in the bible where we misconstrue the meaning of the message in the bible about eating is in Acts 10: 9-16:

> 9. On the morrow, as they went on their journey, and drew nigh unto the city, Peter went up upon the housetop to pray about the sixth hour:
>
> 10. And he became very hungry, and would have eaten: but while they made ready, he fell into a trance,
>
> 11. And saw heaven opened, and a certain vessel descending unto him, as it had been a great sheet knit at the four corners, and let down to the earth:

12. Wherein were all manner of four foot beasts of the earth, and wild beasts, and creeping things, and fowls of the air.

13. And there came a voice to him, Rise, Peter; Kill, and eat.

14. But Peter said, Not so, Lord; for I have never eaten any thing that is common or unclean.

15. And the voice spoke unto him again the second time, What God has cleansed, that call not you common.

16. This was done three thrice: and the vessel was received up again into heaven.

This was a vision that Peter was having. It was not just emphasizing eating foods, but rather Peter going and giving the Word of God (the Gospel) to a Gentiles-which the Jews referred to as dogs or common. Remember, his mission would be to take the Gospel to the Gentile Italian called Cornelius that lived in Caesarea.

The angel was not telling Peter to take Cornelius some food; no, give him the Gospel!

In that same text, you'll note that he did not eat with them; he preached to them, and while he preached to them, the Holy Spirit came on them; so when we try to interpret this text as dealing with us eating anything, we miss the meaning of the entire text.

Whatever laws God instituted still stands, and the Gospel was never intended to cancel out the laws of God.

Jesus makes it plain in Mathew 5: 17-19:

> 17. Think not that I am come to destroy the law, or the prophets: I am not come to destroy, but to fulfill.

> 18. For verily I say unto you, Till heaven and earth pass, one jot or one tittle shall in no wise pass from the law, till all be fulfilled.

> 19. Whosoever therefore shall break one of these least commandments, and shall each men so, he shall be called the least in the kingdom of heaven: but whosoever shall do and teach them, the same shall be called great in the kingdom of heaven.

Jesus was saying that the Gospel was not going to cancel out the laws of God. What God required, He still requires. The Gospel simply helps us meet God's requirements.

We are supposed to stay away from those foods that God calls unclean to us in Leviticus the eleventh chapter. They are not good for us, and give birth to things that are not good for us. They still bring sickness and death.

Some have said, Well, what about what the Apostle Paul says in 1 Timothy 4: 1-5. Note what it says:

> 1. Now the Spirit speaks expressly, that in the latter times some shall depart from the faith, giving heed to seducing spirits, and doctrines of devils;
>
> 2. Speaking lies in hypocrisy; having their conscience seared with a hot iron;
>
> 3. Forbidding to marry, and commanding to abstain from meats, which God has created to be received with thanksgiving of them which believe and know the truth.

4. For every creature of God is good, and
nothing to be refused, if it be received
with thanksgiving:

5. For it is sanctified by the word of God
and prayer.

The Apostle Paul was not giving us a license to eat
anything. He was talking about the hypocrisy that
would come soon-where men of religion would pretend
to fast and abstain from meats.

He says that all creatures of God is good; he is saying
that God created them for a distinct purpose, therefore,
all creatures are good, and none to be frowned upon.

The Apostle Paul was not saying that it is alright for us
to have cock roach and maggots for dinner with a big
helping of flies and boiled mosquitoes on the side. No,
he was pointing out the hypocrisy that was to come by
some religious folks and the future antichrist.

We must eat healthy; that is to say for us to choose
the foods that God designed to help us live long and
healthy lives without being riddled by what man calls
old age.

If we operate within the confines of God's food law, not only will we reap the benefits right now, but our "right eating" will turn around some of our bodily functions that our eating habits had damaged or destroyed.

If you give your body the right foods, it will take care of itself. Just eating is not enough; you've got to eat the right foods, and stay away from the wrong foods.

It's like trying to fill a massive hole with dirt. Yes, you could fill the hole with just a table spoon, but it would take you a hundred years; a shovel would be better, but better still, a bull dozer would do it in just a few hours. Anything that you put in your body will be used for fuel, but it is better to give your body the best foods-the ones that were designed for it.

Remember the old cliché that said that you are what you eat. Yes, it's true; you eat what you are. How do you expect to be healthy when you're eating a sick cow? Whatever sickness the cow has, if you continue eating the cow, you'll have the sickness the cow had; thus, is how people are plagued with high blood pressure, arthritis, gout, allergies, heart disease, and a host of other diseases that eating the wrong foods simply draws to us.

Remember that your body is a temple, a holy temple; and you must treat it as such. You must respect your temple and observe what goes into your temple. Just as in a temple made of mortar and clay that men are very careful what is allowed in the temple -so should it be with your personal temple-your body. Look at what the Apostle Paul says about this matter of your body being a temple. 2 Corinthians 6: 16-18:

16. And what agreement has the temple of God with idols: for you are the temple of the living God; as God has said, I WILL DWELL IN THEM, AND WALK IN THEM; AND I WILL BE THEIR GOD, AND THEY SHALL BE MY PEOPLE.

17. Wherefore COME OUT FROM AMONG THEM, AND BE YOU SEPARATE, says the Lord, AND TOUCH NOT THE UNCLEAN THING; AND I WILL RECEIVE YOU,

18. AND WILL BE A FATHER UNTO YOU, AND YOU SHALL BE MY SONS AND DAUGHTERS, says the Lord Almighty.

The bible is saying that your body is a temple-God's temple, so we should be careful what we allow in our temple. Do not put unclean and defiled things in your temple. REMEMBER, when you put unclean and defiled foods in your body, they attract other things into your body that is not good for you, and brings untimely death and sickness to you.

Note how Jesus referred to His body as a temple. John 2: 19-21:

> 19. Jesus answered and said unto them, Destroy this temple, and in three days I will raise it up.
>
> 20. Then said the Jews, Forty and six years was this temple in building, and will you rear it up in three days?
>
> 21. But he spoke of the temple of his body.

What you must bear to understand is that your body belongs to God; it is where he dwells in you. The unclean foods that you eat (spoken of in Leviticus 11) tares down pollute and slowly tare down your temple.

It is expected of you to live a long and prosperous life because you are connected with The God of the universe. He lives in you-your temple.

Yes, now you understand. Your body is a walking, breathing, moving, active church of the living God.

The bible refers to our bodies as a tabernacle of the living God. A tabernacle is a moving church. It was a tent that could be moved from place to place. Your body is the tabernacle of God-it moves from place to place. Note 2 Corinthians 5: 1-4:

> 1. For we know that if our earthly house of this tabernacle were dis-solved, we have a building of God, an house not made with hands, eternal in the heavens.

> 2. For in this we groan, earnestly desiring to be clothed upon with our house which is from heaven:

> 3. If so be that being clothed with shall not be found naked.

> 4. For we that are in this tabernacle do groan, being burdened: not for that we would be unclothed, but clothed upon,

that mortality might be swallowed up of life.

Our bodies are our church. It is the place that our living God resides. Most Sundays, we take our church to a church made of mortar and clay.

Be very careful what you put into your temple; for it is either prolonging your life, or quickening your death.

The truth of the matter is that we are all going to die some day; for the bible says that it is appointed unto man once to die; so we cannot escape that. But, we are supposed to die of natural causes-just sleep away at a good old healthy age.

All the things that we naturally associate with getting old have much to do with our eating habits than our aging. A woman's hot flashes; a man's erectile dysfunction, we often associate to getting old; and say that a woman's estrogen, and a man's testosterone levels have decreased significantly because of their age, but I submit to you that it has more to do with their diet than growing old. Remember, the bible records that Moses never experienced his body getting old.

Memory lost, Alzheimer, and all the diseases of the mind is do to the effects of a long bad diet filled with unclean defiled foods.

If we stay away from those unclean foods outlined in Leviticus and Deuteronomy, and eat those clean foods also outlined in Leviticus and Deuteronomy, we shall live a long healthy and prosperous life, and when it comes our time to die-as we shall, we shall just sleep away, which man calls dieing of natural causes.

You cannot break God's eating law, and expect to live long and prosperous. When you break God's eating law, you reap the consequences; so when you pick up that spoon or fork, look at what you're about to put into your temple. Is it breaking God's law, or adhering to God's law.

When you're choosing your food from a restaurant's menu, don't break the food law; when you're shopping in the supermarket, don't break the food law; and you shall live a long healthy and prosperous life.

PRAY THIS PRAYER FOR STRENGTH:

Dear heavenly Father, I know your laws that you have established for me. Give me strength now to abide in your laws of life for me. Let me not break your laws so that I can live the life that you ordain for me-to live and not quickly die, or be plagued by sickness and disease that come to all those that will break your laws. Thank you for allowing me to know your laws, acknowledge your laws, and live by your laws-in Jesus name-Amen.

Chapter Six

BY THE SWEAT

**IF MY SEAFOOD DIDN'T HAVE
FINS AND SCALES
IT IS NOT GOOD FOR ME**

To obtain the best health that you can acquire, and walk in the strength of your youth, you've got to sweat!! Look what God said to Adam: Genesis 3: 17-19:

> 17. And unto Adam he said, Because you have hearkened unto the voice of your wife, and have eaten of the tree, of which I commanded you, saying, You shall not eat of it: cursed is the ground for your sake; in sorrow shall you eat of it all the days of your life;

> 18. Thorns also and thistles shall it bring forth to thee; and you shall eat the herb of the field;

> 19. In the sweat of your face shall you eat bread, till you return unto the ground; for out of it were you taken: for dust you are, and unto dust shall you return.

What God was telling us through Adam is that if you want to live and prosper, you've got to do a great degree of sweating-literally sweat; that is why exercise is so beneficial for us because it makes us walk within the confines of God's sentencing for us-you must sweat to live; you must sweat to proper; you must sweat to

maintain good health…sweat…..sweat…..sweat…..
sweat!!!!!

What exactly is sweating???

Sweating is a part of the system that our bodies use to get rid of chemical waste from within our system-other ways are defecation, urination, and exhaling.

The act of sweating also cools the body down. Sweat carries excess heat out of your body and when it evaporates upon your skin, it takes the excess heat with it; thereby cooling the body off, so that one will not suffer from heat stroke, or heat exhaustion.

A person loses weight during sweating because sweat is also the result of fat being burned in the body, and the waste from the fat comes out through your skin's pores; thus, when the fat decreases, the weight of the person decreases.

Also, after we sweat during intense exercise, we have to drink more water and some degree of liquid filled with nutrients because when your body sweats, it not only burns the fat, and get rid of other waste while cooling the body down, it also, at the very same time, gets rid of salt (a very necessary nutrient) and other nutrients in our bodies that we need; which is the reason why sometimes after intense exercise, we will experience some cramps-it is our body's way of telling us and warning us that we need to replenish the nutrients that we expended through our sweat glands because of exercise or whatever intense activity that you have done that caused you to sweat; this is the reason why antiperspirants are not good for us (use deodorant instead). In essence, antiperspirant causes us to stop sweating.

I SHALL EAT RIGHT
I SHALL SWEAT
SO I SHALL LIVE LONG AND PROSPEROUS

Yes, we have to sweat. There is life through the course of sweat. God said that man would live by the sweat of his brow; which means that, to live, and live healthy and prosperous, we have got to sweat; which brings us to **Exercise**.

Exercise is defined as any physical activity that forces your body to burn extra calories-which is where "sweating" comes in. Bottom line is the reason why exercise is so beneficial to you is because it forces you to sweat more; and the more you sweat, the more you expel many of the harmful impurities in your body through your sweat glands.

Exercise heats your body up, and forces many of the organs inside of you to work harder-the definition of getting in shape. Your heart gets stronger because it's forced to work harder; your lungs get stronger because they are forced to inhale and exhale air much faster, and so on, and so on with every body part. When you are sweating, a lot is going on inside of you and out side of you.

Some of the **BENEFITS** of exercising are:

- It decreases the chances of heart disease and stroke

- Helps manage type 1 diabetes, and helps lessen your chances of acquiring type 2 diabetes.
- It helps your body heal faster; a fit body is much more apt to recover faster than one that is out of shape.
- People that regularly exercise are much more likely to be generally happy people because exercise increases the release of some hormones such as dopamine.
- A fit body naturally fights cancer

Exercise, because of all of the above benefits, obviously, helps you to live a longer and healthier life; thereby, rendering you the great possibility of prosperity also.

Note the exercises that produce much sweat and calories burned:

1. Stair climbing, about 1000 calories an hour.
2. Dancing, about 550 calories an hour.
3. Walking at a good pace, about 400 calories an hour.
4. Bicycle riding, about 500 calories an hour.
5. Aerobics, about 550 calories an hour.
6. Swimming, about 1200 calories an hour (swimming burns the most calories because one uses a great deal of muscles when swimming.

7. Basket ball, about 1000 calories an hour.
8. Free weights, about 800 calories an hour.

SWEAT.......SWEAT......SWEAT...... It is God's law given to Adam; "By the sweat of your brow shall you live."

Scientific research says that we have a certain life expectancy. White females often live longer than anyone else. The average Caucasian female's life expectancy is about 80 years; while the African American female's life expectancy is about 75 years. The Caucasian male life expectancy is about 73 years; while the African American life expectancy is about 70 years old.

The reason for this disparity in life expectancy among Caucasians and African Americans is partly because of the difference in their diet, and way of life.

Because we exercise very little, we don't sweat nearly as much as we need to; therefore we are often no where near our supposedly healthy weight class. Notice the weight class that is specified for men and women:

HEIGHT	WEIGHT
4' 11"	95-125
5'0"	97-130

5'1"	100-135
5'2"	108-138
5'3"	110- 145
5'4"	112- 147
5'5"	113-150
5'6"	117-158
5'7"	120-160
5'8"	125-167
5'9"	130-175
5'10"	135-180
5'11"	136-185
6'0"	140-190
6'1"	145-205
6'2	150-210

My weight scale is not consistent with the medical society's suggested weight for men and women; for I am persuaded that their weight suggestion is far too low; particularly for African Americans.

Too, I believe that the scales for which the medical society measures the different numbers for high blood pressure, diabetes glucose, and most other numbers that they weigh to diagnose certain diseases are mostly too low when it comes to African Americans; for their system of experimental measure was performed on mostly Caucasians; therefore, the numbers for tests reflect the result of a Caucasian's system. I believe that

African Americans diagnostic numbers are inherently higher.

No system of good health can be achieved without much sweat- continued sweat from extensive exercise, or work that equals exercise will produce sweat. You cannot get around God's universal law for mankind. He said that we will **LIVE** by **SWEAT!!**

The more that you sweat, the more calories you burn; thereby, causing you to lose those unwanted pounds that's been hanging around your waist or mounted on your buttocks. Note the scale below of how sweating during exercise burns calories of fat:

HOW MANY COLORIES DOES IT TAKE?

Males

Age	Moderate Activity	Intense Activity
20-30	2800-3000 Cals	3000+ Cals
31-45	2200-2600 Cals	2600+ Cals
45+	2200-2400 Cals	2400+ Cals

Females

Age	Moderate Activity	Intense Activity
20-30	2500-2800 Cals	28000+ Cals
31-45	2000-2400 Cals	2400+ Cals
45+	1500-1800 Cals	1800+ Cals

THE ABOVE CHART IS BASED ON MEDIUM HEIGHT AND WEIGHT.

To maintain or lose weight, use the caloric chart above. Lose weight, about a pound a week (it is healthy to lose weight slowly), reduce your daily total calorie intake from the chart by about 500. Thus, you will eat less, and be more active.

If you need to gain weight; use the same scale, but increase your calorie intake by 500, and decrease the intensity of your exercise curriculum.

Early man did not have to go to the gym to sweat and keep in shape. His very existence was exercise that produced sweat. He walked mostly everywhere he needed to go, and worked the fields. He rose up early and worked until late; thus, sweating throughout the day.

Our modern society has hindered us and caused us to sweat less. Our children are more obese mainly because of the gadgets now. They don't readily go out doors and rip and run, or ride their bikes all day; no, they are inside, in air condition playing some kind of game on TV or their phone, or the latest new gadget; so, they are plagued by over weight and obesity.

REMEMBER, sweat is your body's way of cleansing it's system, cooling its self off, and getting rid of some of the impurities in your system; that is why we should avoid antiperspirants, for they stop us from sweating (perspiring) in that spot. We should use simple deodorant instead.

PRAY THIS PRAYER FOR STRENGTH:

Oh my heavenly Father; the God of the entire universe; that made everything that is. I praise you and honor you for making me in your image, and giving me a degree of your strength; that I might have strength over this body that you gave me. Allow me the strength to move my body enough to sweat; let me enjoy exercising enough to sweat. I want to sweat into health, and sweat my unwanted pounds away. Lord give me the wisdom to choose to sweat daily; for I know that in doing so I sweat the impurities out of my body, and sweat my way to a better more healthier life-in Jesus name-Amen.

Chapter Seven

A PARADIGM SHIFT

A paradigm shift, simply put, is to change your concept of things, and the way that you see things. It is a quick change; therefore, paradigm shift is viewed like a revolution-which is a quick devastating change.

The problem with most folks, and the reason why they fail on most diets, is because they want a gradual change. You see, the truth of the matter is that a paradigm shift is often not easy. Most folks cannot just get up one morning and just change their concept of the way that they see things and the world around them. Often times, the problem is not the world around us; many times it is how we see the world around us.

Cakes, candy, pies, cookies, hamburgers, french-fries, and all kinds of sweets, are not our problem; they are harmless and good by themselves. It is when "we" over indulge in these things; when we feel that we cannot help ourselves-we have got to have them, even when our weight is sky rocketing higher, and we are becoming dangerously unhealthy; we still eat them. In other words, we often dig our graves with our appetites.

Remember, a paradigm shift simply means to quickly and suddenly change the way you see and perceive things to be. All of our actions are stimulated by pain and pleasure. The reasons why we do what we do are motivated by pain and pleasure.

So, in order for us to have a successful paradigm shift, we must shift our level of pain and pleasure for certain things. Candy, cookies, pies, hamburgers, french-fries, and all those other sweets and high calorie foods, you have got to associate them with much pain and displeasure. You've got to become disgusted with the weight that you have gained, and have no pleasure with being over weight, and eating those foods that are not good for you; such as pork and all the other unclean foods that God told us not to eat.

You must find pleasure in the foods that are good for you, and produce good health; find pleasure in looking good and being shapely and toned. You must find pleasure in exercising and working-out.

Unless you associate much pain and much pleasure to your situation, you're unlikely to change for very long; that's why just dieting is not enough-you've got to have a paradigm shift-you've got to suddenly and quickly change the way that you see things and yourself; become disgusted with "you", so that you can foster the pleasure of a **new you.**

Our societies are accustomed to paradigm shifts. We just don't call what has taken place as a paradigm shift, but that is exactly what has happened.

One of the greatest paradigm shifts in the world happened in the East-in Israel. Jesus ushered in a paradigm shift to the world of religion-particularly to the Jews.

Jesus explains the paradigm shift in the bible in the book of Matthew; note what he says: Matthew 5: 21-45:

> 21. You have heard that it was said by them of old time, you shall not kill; and whosoever shall kill shall be in danger of the judgment:

> 22. But I say unto you, That whosoever is angry with his brother without a cause shall be in danger of the judgment: and whosoever shall say to his brother, Raca, shall be in danger of the council: but whosoever shall say, You fool, shall be in danger of hell fire.

> 23. Therefore if you bring your gift to the altar, and there remember that your brother has ought against you;

24. Leave there your gift before the altar, and go your way; first be reconciled to your brother, and then come and offer your gift.

25. Agree with your adversary quickly, whiles you are in the way with him; lest at any time the adversary deliver you to the officer, and you be cast into prison.

26. Verily I say unto you, you shall by no means come out there, till you have paid the uttermost farthing.

27. You have heard that it was said by them of old time, You shall not commit adultery:

28. But I say unto you, That whosoever looks on a woman to lust after her has committed adultery with her already in his heart.

29. And if your right eye offend you, pluck it out, and cast it from you: for it is profitable for you that one of your members should perish, and not that your whole body should be cast into hell.

30. And if your right hand offend you, cut it off, and cast it from you: for it is profitable for you that one of your members should perish, and not that your whole body should be cast into hell.

31. It has been said, Whosoever shall put away his wife, let him give her a writing of divorcement:

32. But I say unto you, That whosoever shall put away his wife, saving for the cause of fornication, causes her to commit adultery: and whosoever shall marry her that is divorced commits adultery.

33. Again, you have heard that it has been said by them of old time, You shall not forswear yourself, but shall perform unto the Lord your oaths:

34. But I say unto you, Swear not at all; neither by heaven; for it is God's throne:

35. Nor by the earth; for it is his footstool: neither by Jerusalem; for it is the city of the great King.

36. Neither shall you swear by your head, because you cannot make one hair white or black.

37. But let your communication be, Yes, yes; No, no: for whatsoever is more than these comes of evil.

38. You have heard that it has been said, an eye for an eye, and a tooth for a tooth:

39. But I say unto you, That you resist not evil: but whosoever shall smite you on your right cheek, turn to him the other also.

40. And if any man will sue you at the law, and take away your coat, let him have your cloke also.

41. And whosoever shall compel you to go a mile, go with him two.

42. Give to him that asks you, and from him that would borrow of you turn not you away.

43. You have heard that it has been said, You shall love your neighbor, and hate your enemy.

44. But I say unto you, Love your enemies, bless them that curse you, do good to them that hate you, and pray for them which despitefully use you, and persecute you;

45. That you may be the children of your Father which is in heaven: for he makes his sun to rise on the evil and on the good, and sends rain on the just and on the unjust.

What Jesus was introducing his disciples to was a paradigm shift-new concepts in the way that they had been viewing things, and a new way of believing; That is why the old Judaic priests hated Jesus-he was causing the people to see things differently, and change their mental concept of what God and religion was.

It was not the secular world that crucified Jesus; it was formal religious leaders who coerced the Romans to crucify him.

Even now, most of the world is affected by Jesus' introduction of a paradigm shift over two thousand years ago. It is called Christianity. It gives new concepts to God in relationships, forgiveness, righteousness, heaven, and hell.

If you don't like what you see, then, change the way that you see it. You must see the importance of eating the right foods, and reframing from the unhealthy.

I know that it is difficult and painful; real change is always accompanied by difficulty and pain; that's why most people choose not to change. But, when you become disgusted with back problems, knee problems, ankle problems, shortness of breath, arthritis, heart problems, diabetes, and a host of other problems that are associated with over weight and obesity, you will choose to have a paradigm shift.

We see shifts in patterns of thinking all the time through out history. The United States were force to embrace a paradigm shift as a nation when it came to slavery. They began to see human commodity as indecent, wrong, and inhumane. A painful war ensued because our nation had a mental shift in how they saw slavery in 1865.

What caused many of the Jim Crow laws to change in the South is because the world started seeing the ugliness and shamefulness of segregation. It embarrassed us as a nation around the world (caused our nation much pain), so we had a paradigm shift and developed new laws.

In order for you to be successful in this new diet, to create a new and healthier you, you have got to shift the way that you have been seeing yourself, and see the new you; and you must, right now, become disgusted with your weight and potentially unhealthy disposition.

PRAY THIS PRAYER FOR STRENGTH:

Lord, I know that I need a paradigm shift in my life right now, for my old way of thinking has brought me sickness, death, and unhappiness. Give me the strength to thinking differently, and to see things differently. Give me the strength to walk away from those things that I need to walk away from, and the strength to put off those things that I need to cut off. Master, let me see and walk in new life; that I might come forth a new and strong person that is willing to do what it takes to live a long, prosperous, healthy, and joy filled life-in Jesus name-Amen.

Chapter Eight

EATING TO PERFORM

How many times have you turned your T.V on late at night to some man or woman on the screen with a host of other folks telling you of how much weight they have lost- Individual after individual telling you, and showing you before and after pictures of how much weight that they have lost?

A man or woman comes on the screen with their midsections cut like a washboard, and their arms and legs tight and toned. They guarantee you through the T.V that you can lose weight and be cut just like them; often times, they give you this exercise program that is usually too good to be true (My granddaddy said that if it sounds like it is too good to be true, then it usually is). One such program, told the viewers that all they would have to do is just exercise hard for thirty minutes each day-exercises that drenched your body in sweat and fatigue. Truthfully, yes, if you do those strenuous exercises every day, you will lose weight. The problem is, how many of us are going to continue on such an exercise regimen for very long, not to mention doing it for the rest of our lives.

On the other hand, there are these diets, too, that are advertised that is simply too farfetched to achieve any degree of long term effect on weight lost and health; like the all protein diet, or the cut out all carbohydrates, or what about the no sugar diet, and last, but not least, just fasting and not eating at all for days at a time. All of the fore mentioned diets always fail and have no long term healthy weight lost effect. Most participants lose, but end up gaining all the weight that they lost back, and usually gain a few pounds more.

You must acquire a program that is right for you and is also good for your system. It matters little if you lose weight but become sick from the methods by which you lost.

Your system has to have balance. God created us to have balance right down to our very cellular level. It is called osmosis. Too much sugar is not good for you, but no sugar at all is just as bad; sugar is so needed in your diet until God created most eatable things with a degree of sugar in them. There has to be **BALANCE** in our diets.

The primary reason why we eat is to gain fuel to do work. Food is our fuel like gas to a car. The more fuel you acquire, the more work that you can do-work is anything that the body physically do; even a body at rest requires a certain degree of fuel to function. While lying still, your body is still at work keeping everything in your system functioning-circulating the blood, pumping the heart, filtering the kidneys, etc.

The problem arise when we take in more food fuel than we need for work, therefore, our bodies store the excess intake-turning it into fat, thus, is the reason why we have over weight and obese people.

Simply put, if you want to lose weight, you must burn more fuel than you take in, for just as the body stores fuel when it has enough to perform the work at hand, it also burns some of that stored fuel (fat) when it has not taken in enough to perform the work at hand-thus, causing the body to lose weight.

Yes, those late night advertisements for exercise CDs that shows you how to work your body hard for 30 minutes can work, but truthfully, how many of us are going to work to that intensity for the rest of our lives, or even for a few years? None of us; so you must do something that is practical for you and your body.

You have to consider many variables when determining to lose weight; such as your height, family history, genetics, etc. God didn't create all of us to be a size 2, or 6, and He didn't create all of us to be big boned with big statues.

We must start eating to live, and not living to eat. We have to eat to be able to perform our daily task, but remember, when we take in more than needed for our daily task, the body stores it as fat.

Balancing what you eat; this is where we get the phrase **nutritional health** from. Nutrition simply defined is the process of providing or obtaining the food necessary for health and growth-to have good health and grow, you must have a nutritiously balanced diet-not too much sugar, not too much protein, not too much carbohydrates, but balanced.

Good nutrition is your best friend for good health! Poor nutrition sabotages your attempt to good health even when you're exercising with great intensity. Eating the right foods at the right time gives you optimum health; that is why in previous chapters we discussed the importance of plenty of fruits and vegetables in your diet. Your intake of the right foods will help your body naturally heal itself, and help you acquire the rest and recovery that you need after any work have been done. Bad nutrition leads to bad health.

To eat for performance, or work, or whatever it is that you do, you must have a degree of good nutrition. Breakfast, lunch and dinner with healthy snacks in between are very important to good health, and even losing weight. Sometimes, we defeat ourselves on our weight lost diets by restricting ourselves from eating.

Eating is not your problem; your problem is **"when"** you eat, and **"what"** you eat when you eat.

Three healthy meals a day and healthy snacks in between will produce good health. Your nutritional intake should be balanced with carbohydrates, proteins, and fats. About fifty percent of your daily intake should come from complex carbohydrates; twenty percent from fat and three percent of the fat should come from unsaturated fat which is gained from such foods as oils and plants. Unsaturated fat, unlike saturated fat, remains in a liquid form in room temperature; which is the reason people consuming a lot of saturated fat gain weight-Fat is the last food to leave the stomach, which gives the body a slow feeling of satisfaction; thus, acquiring a feeling to desire more food before the 'I am satisfied' feeling comes on, which in tern, leads to weight gain and obesity.

About fifteen percent of your diet should be filled with protein. Protein functions throughout your body; it is essential in building muscle, helping replace old cells, helping to vitalize nails, skin, and hair among so many other functions of the body.

If we balance our nutritional intake, we will live healthier lives. Remember, three healthy meals a day with healthy snacks in between will produce a healthy vibrant body. Your diet should be mostly complex carbohydrates-which are from foods such as whole grain, pasta, fruit (raw), and vegetables, potatoes, and rice. Simple carbohydrates should be avoided; for they, unlike complex carbohydrates, inter your system quickly and raise your blood glucose level quickly, but don't last long, so they require the individual to have to eat more simple carbohydrates to sustain that energy level; too, when the simple carbohydrate diminishes, they often leaves the individual drained and low of energy which makes the individual not apt to want to exercise for lack of energy-thus, requiring the person to replenish themselves with more simple carbohydrates. Some of the simple carbohydrates are candy, table sugar, jams, jellies, soft drinks, fruit juices, table and other syrups, products made with white flour-white bread, white pasta, cakes, pastries, packaged cereal, sucrose, fructose, and processed, refined sugars; these are the ones you really want to stay away from, or not eat as often. Some fruit have simple carbohydrate, but are also rich in vitamins, so I don't recommend abstaining from fruits. Their benefits far out weight their detriment.

To eat to perform, we must eat smaller meals and eat often. This keeps your metabolism continuously burning calories; too, remember that fat has twice the calories in it as the same amount of protein or carbohydrate, so be careful of your fat intake.

Also, I must admit that there is a distinct place for simple carbohydrates. They are good for when you have exerted yourself to exhaustion, and you have used all of your energy (glucose), and you feel like you can go no further, for your energy in depleted. Simple carbohydrates can reboot your energy levels fast; and often times without that "filled up and full" sensation.

To get the most out of your daily work and to perform at your best, you must eat the right foods. Remember to watch **"what"** you eat, and **"when"** you eat. I recommend that you eat nothing after seven o'clock in the evening-particularly anything heavy.

Remember also, to achieve the most from your diet, you must also allow yourself proper rest and sleep. Rest and sleep is when your body go to work at repairing and restoring whatever your daily work has damaged.

If you watch what you eat, you should be able to live a long and healthy life that is able to perform any task at hand.

Be patient with yourself, for a life time of eating wrong and eating all the time all the wrong foods does not change over night; to think so, is setting yourself up for failure. It can become unhealthy to lose more than two pounds a week. Any amount more puts a degree of unhealthy stress upon your body.

The slower that you lose weight, the more apt you are to keeping it off, and vise versa, the quicker that you take the unwanted weight off, the quicker you put it back on, and usually, you put on more weight.

- Always consult your doctor before any plan of substantial weight loss.
- Three healthy meals with healthy stacks in between-five smaller portioned meals a day.
- Watch your carbohydrates, and reframe as much as possible from simple carbohydrates such as candy, fruit juice, syrup, sodas, and Jams and jellies, white breads, and white pastas.
- Make sure you consume a good degree of protein in your diet; this helps your body repair, maintain and rebuild itself.
- Never skip breakfast. It jumpstarts your metabolism.
- Fill your day with prayer to succeed. In order to change your way of living, you need to believe in a higher power-something that's greater than yourself.

PRAY THIS PRAYER FOR STRENGTH

Dear heavenly Father, oh good and most gracious Jehovah, give me the strength this day to adhere to a diet that will produce positive results in my body so that I can perform the daily tasks that I have declared for myself, and the things that You have commissioned me to do; I pray that you would grant me with health and strength as you have blessed so many of your servants in the past. Thank you right now for I believe that it is already done; I receive your blessing of strength to change my way of eating and mind-set so that now I eat to live, and not live to eat. In Jesus name I pray-Amen.

Chapter Nine

FASTING

Give your system a rest

In its simplest form, fasting means to abstain from all or some kinds of food or drink, especially as a religious observance.

Fasting is just as necessary to the body as the intake of food; the bible commands us to fast often.

Note what Jesus says of us fasting: Luke 5:35:

> 35: But the days will come, when the bridegroom shall be taken away from them, and then shall they fast in those days.

Jesus said that His followers would fast. He didn't say that it would be good for them to fast; no, he said that they would fast-period.

You see, fasting does essentially two things:

1. Fasting allows your body to rest and get rid of a lot of the toxins that have been stored up in your system-such as your digestive system. It allows the digestive system to cleanse itself-to get rid of some of those food particles that has been attached to your digestive wall for too long. Your system gets a good "flush" out. During fasting, it also begins to eat some of that stored up fat that you've been carrying too long.

CHOOSE TO LIVE
AND YOU WILL LIVE TO CHOOSE

In nature, many animals that live a long life, often go weeks without eating-naturally fasting.

2. Fasting gives us spiritual resolve; it strengthens our spiritual man. During your fast, you are denying yourself food while praying and seeking directions from God; that's why Jesus told His disciples to fast-because you need God's voice, God's guidance, and God's power to fulfill what He has called you to do.

Fasting weakens our physical person while, at the very same time strengthening our spiritual person-making you weak physically (for a moment), but increasing your strength spiritually.

For now, though, we are focusing on fasting's physical aspect upon the body-cleansing the body.

All of us innately fast every day. It is when we sleep; we are fasting overnight-that is why the first meal that we eat in the morning is called breakfast-break-fast. In other words, when you awaken in the morning and eat, you are breaking the fast that you were on last night.

Whether it is two days, three days, or several weeks, you must force yourself to fast.

Do not start out trying to go several days if you are not accustom to fasting. Start with a half a day, then one day, then two days and so forth.

Simpler than that is to perhaps restrict "what" you eat until you can acquire enough strength to abstain from all foods for a period of time; such as eating only vegetables.

The famous Daniel fast is eating only vegetables for a given period of time. Note what the bible says about Daniel's fast. Daniel 1: 11-15:

> 11: Then said Daniel to Melzar: whom the prince of the eunuchs had set over Daniel, Hananiah, Mishael, and Azariah,

> 12: Prove your servants, I beseech you, ten days; and let them give us pulse to eat, and water to drink.

> 13: Then let our countenances be looked upon before you, and the countenance of the children that eat of the portion of the king's meat: and as you see, deal with your servants.

14: So he consented to them in this matter, and proved them ten days.

15: And at the end of ten days their countenances appeared fairer and fatter in flesh than all the children which did eat the portion of the king's meat.

In this scripture of Daniel's fast, pulse, simply means vegetables. In other words, Daniel and his friends fasted for ten days eating vegetables only, and drinking only water.

Note in verse 15, it says that they looked fairer than the others who were eating the meat. Their skin looked better and fuller-better than those that were eating the meat.

Thus, is where we acquired our "Daniel Fast".

I simply emphasize that you must include some degree of fasting in your diet routine!!

* **Fast regularly**
* **Fast intently**
* **Fast purposely**

PRAY THIS PRAYER FOR STRENGTH:

Dear Heavenly Father I thank you right now for giving me the strength to fast often and reap the benefits of fasting. Thank you for new extended life. I honor you with this improve healthy body of mind.

In Jesus name I pray-Amen

Chapter Ten

EAT TO LIVE

You should always be very aware of what you are putting in your mouth; knowing full well that everything that goes into your mouth has a great affect upon your body; which is why you should choose carefully what you eat. I believe that man can easily live to be two hundred, or three hundred years if he chooses very carefully what he puts in his mouth.

He must eat the right portions of the right foods; else he slowly kills himself with his spoon.

Remember, you live and are nourished by your caloric intake. Your diet is giving you life, or bringing you death. In this chapter, we are attempting to show some foods that we need to be sure to include in our diets, and some to restrict in our diets. Exercise alone is not enough to warrant long life; we must also eat right.

There are six essential nutrients that our bodies must have to have adequate life; they are:

1. Water
2. Fat
3. Protein
4. Carbohydrates
5. Vitamins
6. Minerals

An essential nutrient is a nutrient that the body cannot make on its on, or it makes too little to sustain adequate body function.

Let's take a look at each of them individually and see what is their function in the body.

1. Water- It helps to maintain homeostasis (balance inside and outside the wall of the cell) in the body. We should drink one to two liters of water a day; though we don't have to consume our water intake just in the liquid form; there are some foods that are high in water. Believe it or not, you can consume too much water; too much, flushes out some of the nutrients that you need; it will flush out a lot of your salt intake, and potassium, etc. You have to be careful not to consume too much water. We must be careful to keep ourselves hydrated inside and out. Proper skin care is saturated with plenty of water.

2. Fat-Although most diets warn you to keep away from fats, fat is a very necessary part of our diet; not enough fat in your diet can produce an unhealthy body. Basically, fat is a long term energy source for your body. It increases the absorption of fat-soluble vitamins like vitamins A, E, and D. Twenty to twenty-five percent of your daily caloric intake should come from fat;

too, you must choose healthy fats-not all fats are good for you. The healthy fats are that which is found in Omega-3 rich foods. Omega-3 fatty acids play an important role in maintaining the health of the brain as well as protection against certain forms of cancer. Some of the best sources of omega-3 is from cold water fatty fish like wild salmon and mackerel. Some other foods that are high in omega-3 are flaxseed, wheat germ, walnuts, soybeans, mango, deep green leafy vegetables, bluefish, halibut, and tuna. Research says that omega-3 fights coronary heart disease, depression, anxiety, and help with wound healing.

3. Protein- Protein is responsible for the building and repair of body tissue. It is the building blocks of the body. It helps to regenerate the cell. Between fifteen and thirty-five percent of your caloric intake should be protein; for the body constantly needs new cells (old age is simply the cells has stopped regenerating themselves). A good source of protein can be gotten largely from meats, dairy, and eggs. You can also purchase high protein powder drink mixes from your local health food store.

4. Carbohydrates- Carbohydrates are the main energy source of the brain. When we take in more than what we need for our brain and other

functions, our bodies store it; thus, producing over-weigh and obesity. Some of the main sources of carbohydrates are fruits, potatoes, pasta, grains, vegetables, and, of course, sugars. If you want to lose weight, limit your intake of carbohydrates; that is usually anything that is white-potatoes, rice, bread...etc.

5. Vitamins- Vitamins are essential for human maintenance and development. They assist in keep the body in balance, and assist in all the organs and cells work together. Some of the rich vitamins are A, E, C, D, and K.

6. Minerals- Minerals assist in a host of bodily function, and keep the body performing the tasks it needs to do work to survive. Some of the minerals are salt, calcium, and potassium.

If we eat the six essential nutrients daily, and not be gluttons, we would live a healthy sick free life. We would need doctors visits less and less; though I think that everybody ought to be examined once a year by their doctor.

We must strive to have a balanced diet of protein, carbohydrates, fats (particularly omega-3 fatty acids), etc. Remember, all foods have their place if taken in moderation; complex carbohydrates, simple carbohydrates, and sugars, all have their place and was designed for certain purposes; like simple carbohydrates design is to give you a quick burst of energy, but if too much is consumed, then the body stores it and you carry it around your waist or on your thighs as fat.

We need to eat smaller portions more regularly-eat about five times a day.

If you are dieting and eating only one meal a day, or if you are just consuming little or no calories-like eating only lettuce, then you won't lose at all, or lose very little because the body is designed to preserve itself; so when it is not getting enough calories, it goes into preservation mode and store up fat and slows down its metabolism -thus making you not lose at all, or very little.

It was God's designed for man, His creation, to live a long and prosperous life, but when he started to eating the wrong foods, man decreased his life expectancy substantially. As fore mentioned, I believe that with the right diet and right living and exercise, man can still live to be two and three hundred years old..

Compared to the longevity of life that man used to have, like Methuselah 969 years old, man now dies young, like little children- He rarely reaches the age of 100; at the beginning of creation, man rarely died before he was in his hundreds.

Remember, there is purpose to your eating, and it is not merely to satisfy your taste buds. Eating is the method by which we fuel our bodies to do work; it is suppose to give us life. But, when we eat the wrong foods, it enters us and began to destroy us from the inside out. What we eat is either giving us extended life, or quickened death.

Many of our diseases can be gotten rid of by our diet-high blood pressure, type 2 diabetes, gout, arthritis, migraine head aches, allergies, cancer, heart disease, ninety percent of them are because of our diets.

If we eat to live, and not live to eat, we will live longer and more fulfilling lives.

God has already done the work for us. The foods that he created to help us live and repair our failing parts he made them to look like what they would help. Notice, when you cut open a tomato, it looks just like our heart's design; walnuts and pecans look like our brains; figs look like our groin; so on and so forth. Many of our foods are in the image of our body parts, which leads me to believe that those foods are designed to help the body part that it looks like….the liver, the pancreas, the kidneys, the heart, the brain, all have fruits or vegetables that image them; which I believe is God's way of giving us some clue which foods are good for which parts of our bodies, particularly if we are having problems with that part.

It is God's desire for us to live, prosper, and be in good health. The Bible reflects this principal very clearly in the book of 3 John 1:2:

> 2. Beloved, I wish above all things that you may prosper and be in health, even as your soul prospers.

The Apostle John was saying that he desired that we have prosperity and good health even as our souls do. In

**DO NOT JUST LIVE TO EAT
BUT EAT TO LIVE
AND WATCH THE NEW VIBRANT YOU
COME FORTH**

other words, he is saying that our souls are sure and safe because God is the watcher and keeper of our souls; and just like our souls are sure and good, our bodies and our daily living should be good.

This only happens when we make a conscious effort to change our lives for the better, and start living as we were designed to live. Eating right is included in change; for if we don't change the way that we eat, then we can be prosperous, but not be able to fully enjoy our prosperity.

Your change of life style of eating right and selecting the right foods that will increase your life will not just happen. It will not just serendipitously happen; you will not stumble into it. You have got to consciously choose and decide to change your life. God will not do that for which you can do for yourself!

Your present diet is designed to kill you and rob you of life. **YOU ARE SUPPOSED TO LIVE A FULL LIFE!!!**

Look what Jesus said about us living; John 10:10:

10. The thief comes not, but for to steal, and to kill, and to destroy: I am come that they might have life, and that they might have it more abundantly.

YOU ARE SUPPOSED TO LIVE!!

YOU ARE GOING TO LIVE!!!

LIVE!!

LIVE!!

LIVE!!

You keep declaring this even if right now you don't believe that you have the strength to achieve this; keep saying it until you can believe it, and soon you shall find yourself with strength to achieve it. **YOU SHALL LIVE AND NOT DIE!!!**

Choose to live, and you will live to choose!

PRAY THIS PRAYER FOR STRENGTH.......

Oh Heavenly Father, Great God Jehovah, I thank you for exposing me to this knowledge of how to eat right and eat to live a long life as you have purposed for me in the beginning when you created me. Now Father give me the strength to change my eating habits so that I shall live and not die. Give me the Godly wisdom to select those foods that you created for me. Open my spiritual eyes that I might see what you have designed that's best for me, and I will give you all the glory and honor. I claim life, health, and strength right now; in Jesus name I pray....Amen.

Chapter Eleven

THE IMPORTANCE OF EXERCISE

Fit for life

Our lives today are designed to kill us and shorten our life. During the earlier days, we didn't have to tell our forefathers to eat right and exercise so that they could prolong their lives. They ate as God had directed, and they did not have to do exercise as we presently know it because their daily lives were filled with exercise.

Our forefathers usually walked where they needed to go, and they did very laborious work. They worked from sun up until sun down-stretching, pulling, lifting, holding, and standing for endless hours. Hard labor was apart of the daily lives, so their work gave them all the exercise that they needed.

The reason why I say that we have death by design is because our society is readily prepared for us to eat all the wrong foods; foods that are simply lethal for us in the long run; all the fast food restaurants with the fat filled hamburgers, greasy French fries, and sugar laden soft drinks, pies and ice cream, are sending a great many of us to the grave on a fast paste roller coaster.

The United States leads the way among nations of the world in obesity.

Most of our high tech gadgets are not designed to entice us to exercise. We drive everywhere that we need to go, even if it is right down the street. Our children do not play like they use to. The video games, phones, television, and X boxes have made them become stationary and only exercise their fingers while their bodies become stricken with obesity.

When we go shopping, or to the grocery store, we want to park as close to the front door as possible because we don't like to walk.

But, we must change if we want to live. It is not enough just to change our diets and choose to eat right, but we must include exercise in our daily routine. Work those muscles to get that atrophy out. The more that you work your muscles, the leaner and stronger they become.

The biggest misconception that most of us have is that the medical world is trying to heal us; they don't want the masses to get completely healed-just get better enough to keep coming to the doctor, or keep getting their treatment.

If the medical world healed all the people that they could, they would simply lose money. They could no longer sell their medicine, or give those expensive treatments. No, they have a billion dollar industry that needs you to be sick. They are not about to show you how they can make less money; they are not about to let their stocks fall. They want, no, they need for you to remain sickly; that's how they make their money and pay their bills-how else can a pharmacist justify charging several hundred dollars to several thousand dollars for a few pills.

You have got to choose to live and be healthier; and including exercise in daily life is the right choice.

You must first start your exercise routine slow, very slow. If you try to go too fast, you're going to do too much, and then quit because you are too sore (soreness is your body signaling you that you have over worked it, and it needs rest, or else injury will ensue. Let it rest!) ; so start slowly and work your way up to more strenuous exercises later.

Remember, one step at a time. You did not get in such bad shape over night, and you will not get into good shape over night.

To lose weight, you must coordinate your eating habits with your food consumption. You can exercise all day, and still gain weight, or not lose a pound, if you are taking in more than you are burning up. In other words, if you go to the gym, and you only burn 1500 calories during your work out, and after the work out, you consume 3000 calories, then you will gain because you have taken in an excess amount of 1500 calories.

Make everything an exercise! When you go to the shopping mall, park as far away from the front door as you possibly can-Thereby, forcing yourself to walk further. Always take the stairs instead of the elevator when possible.

When sitting at your desk, grab the arms of your chair while still sitting, and push yourself up, then ease yourself back down, and slowly push back up again until you can't do any more. This simple exercise is good for your arms and shoulders.

Stand up at your desk, and do half squats starting off; do as many as you can. Eventually, you will be able to do full squats. This will help tone your thighs and give you over-all body strength.

Stand flat footed, then tip toe on the ball of your feet over and over again-up and down, up and down; until your calves burn. This will help tone your calves.

Roll your neck around your shoulders for a minute, then stretch both your arms out to your side, level with your shoulders, and make big circular motions;

as you get tired, make your circular motions smaller and smaller until you can do no more.

Stand a few feet in front of your desk, and place the palms of your hands on the edge of your desk, and do half push ups from this position. Do a couple of sets; like three sets of ten-this will tone your chest.

When at home, lie on your back and raise your knees, and tuck your chin into your chest with your hands behind your head; raise your upper torso up to a forty-five degree angle and hold it for five seconds, and then slowly lower yourself back to the floor. Repeat this for ten times. This is good for your stomach.

In the morning, before you go to work, take you a brisk walk; not only is it good exercise for you, but those early morning ions in the air will do your lungs and body good.

If you can, get you a partner to exercise with you; for you will be much more successful with your workout routine if you have a partner. You will be less apt to quit because someone else is watching you and expecting you to complete the task.

If you can, join a gym because you will be more prone to exercise among others who are endeavoring to exercise. Do not join a gym where everybody in there is buffed up; you will soon become intimidated and cease to go work out.

And remember, before you leave the house for work, breakfast is just as important as exercise-it cranks up your metabolism.

Remember, you are not going to stick with those televisions high intensity exercise gurus. Choose something that you can stick to, something that will foster long term success.

So often, the greatest challenge is not losing the weight, it is keeping it off. Many times, some will lose the weight, but can't keep it off. They often weigh back all that they lost, plus a few extra pounds.

Through daily exercise, you also learn how to minimize your stress, which is also bad for your health.

God built in us a "good" stress mechanism. It is the fight or flight syndrome. When we get in trouble, or danger is upon us, our stress level rises and gives us the ability to run or fight.

Every animal has this; the difference is, in the animal kingdom, they recover as they are supposed to. If a car or an elephant is about to run over them, or if they are threatened by another animal, their stress mechanism engages and gives them that extra ordinary strength for self-preservation-fight or run.

The difference between man and the animal is that ninety seconds after the animal's ordeal has passed, their stress level goes back to normal. They are no longer in their fight or run intensified mode.

However, after man's immediate intensified stress ordeal has ended, unlike the animal's ninety seconds back to normal state, man often chooses to remain in that state-being angry and upset for days, even months over what somebody has done to them, or tried to do to them.

You must learn how to let it go. It's not that deep! Do this breathing exercise every day to help you learn how to de-stress yourself.

Stand with your feet shoulder length apart, with your arms hanging to your side; or if you are sitting, rest your hands in your lap.

Slowly take a deep breath. Slowly fill your lungs and your stomach with fresh new air. You should see your stomach slowly expand outwardly just as your chest does too; then slowly, very slowly exhale-noticing your stomach and chest deflating slowly. Close your eyes and allow yourself to mentally go some place wonderful that you have visited before. If you have gone to Hawaii, imagine yourself there now; hear the waves beating upon the beach. Where ever peaceful place you have gone to in the past, allow yourself to mentally go there while you are doing this breathing exercise.

Perform this exercise a couple of times a day to learn how to de-stress and handle your daily stress.

When you become comfortable doing this exercise, you can over and over again, at a moment's gesture of stress or bad negative drama began letting your mind go off to those wonderful places that you visited and enjoyed in the past; yes, maybe back to some beach, or island, or some city, or some moments that you spent laughing and loving with your love ones. Whatever it takes to ease your mind and lower your stress mood, then ease into that place during your breathing exercise.

Exercise does little good, if you don't change your mental capacity.

I also emphasize the importance of rest between bouts of exercise. You must always allow your body to recover from exercise; or else your exercise can result in injury. When resting, the body restores and recovers from your day's labor-be it exercise or just general work-not getting enough rest, put added stress upon the body, and defeats all that you have done exercising earlier; so be sure to get the proper rest that you need-six to eight hours of sleep every night; sometimes more, depending upon how hard you worked prior to journeying to rest, but you should always get at least six hours of restful sleep!

Chapter Twelve

CHOOSING THE RIGHT MEALS

**BUFFETS AND ALL YOU CAN
EAT RESTAURANTS
ARE YOUR ENEMIES
THEY ENTICE YOU TO OVEREAT**

What we choose to eat, is an attempt to fill our body's nutritional needs. Nutrition is fuel for our bodies to do work. We all need some carbohydrates, some proteins, and some fats, which all come from the foods that we eat; thus is the reason why some of us have poor nutritional habits. We don't select a healthy diet.

Sometimes we can eat too much protein, too much carbohydrates, and too much fat which produces an unhealthy life riddled with sickness and disease. Basically, we all have the same nutritional needs-some things we need a little more than others, depending upon our age and conditions.

When we eat our meals, we should have a dietary nutritional plate as recommended by the USDA; that means that our dinner plate should be broken down into good nutritional portions for us-small portions, I stress. If you cannot see any of the bottom of your plate, your portions are probably too large. You can eat the right food, but too large a portions defeats the purpose; remember, everything that your body doesn't need for energy, it stores it as fat.

Our plate should consist of at least three (we should get all five during our day) of the five essential nutrients that our body needs in some form or other; they are:

1. **fruits**
2. **vegetables**
3. **grain**
4. **protein**
5. **dairy**

These five foods are the building blocks to a healthy diet.

Fruits are any kind of fruit, and 100% fruit juice also counts as fruit. They can be fresh or canned, although I personally feel like fresh is much better for you than canned, frozen, or dried; and it doesn't matter whether it is whole, cut, or mixed.

Fruits are of all different sorts; they include, but not limited to, berries, melons, and 100% fruit juices-fruits like apples, bananas grapes oranges peaches plums tangerines, apricots, cherries, grapefruits, pineapples, etc. (Be aware that too much fruit will give you too much fructose-fruit sugar).

Vegetables are all vegetables including 100% vegetable juice; most are best when they are lightly cooked-still a little crispy. Fresh Vegetables are best, but they can be frozen, canned, or dried.

Vegetables are Dark green, Beans and peas, Starchy, and Red and Orange.

Some of the vegetables are: Mustard greens collard greens broccoli, romaine lettuce, spinach, corn field peas black eyed peas, green peas, potatoes, black beans, kidney beans, beets, cabbage, celery, green peppers, lettuce, okra mushrooms, soy beans, cucumbers, carrots, sweet potatoes, squash, ect.

Grains are any foods made whom wheat, rice, oats, cornmeal, barley, and any other made of the grain products.

Grains are divided into two groups; they are **Whole** Grains and **Refined** Grains.

Examples of Whole Grains are Whole wheat flour, oat meal, whole cornmeal, and brown rice.

Examples of Refined grains are simply grains that have been milled (a process that removes the bran and germ; this gives grains a finer texture, but it also removes some things that our body needs; such as fiber, iron, and many B vitamins.

Some examples of Refined Grain products are: White bread, de-germ corn meal, white bread and white rice.

Dairy is all fluid milk products and many foods made from milk are considered part of the dairy food group. Most Dairy groups choices should be fat-free or low-fat. The dairy food group is rich in calcium. Foods made from milk that has little or no calcium are not considered of the dairy food group; such as cream, butter, and cream cheese.

As we stated before, you should choose fat-free or low-fat dairy products because dairy of it self is high in fat, and too much fat is not good for your health-even though we need some portions of fat in our diets, still, we must choose carefully and monitor our fat intake carefully.

Some dairy products are: skim milk, low fat milk reduced fat milk, whole milk, chocolate milk, lactose reduced milk, and lactose free milk, hard natural cheese, Swiss and cheddar, mozzarella, parmesan, soft cheeses, ricotta, cottage, American cheese, yogurt, milk based desserts, puddings, ice milk, frozen yogurt ice cream, and soy beverages.

The foods that we choose can either bring us good health or poor health; and too much of any one food group can be unhealthy for you; you must acquire balance in your diet.

So often, it is not what you eat, but how much and how often you eat it; sometimes portions are everything.

We should eat like a bird-small portions often; about five meals a day; this will keep your metabolism burning continuously.

Too much of some foods can be unhealthy for us, but in small portions, and not so often, they can also give us good health.

For instance, too much of some foods raise your cholesterol. There are two kinds of cholesterol -LDL (low-density lipoprotein) and HDL (High-density lipoprotein). Cholesterol is a type of fat found in your body.

LDL is called bad cholesterol because it can build up in the walls of your arteries and form plague (get hard), and plague build up in your arteries interfere with blood flow, which increases your risk of heart disease.

HDL is called good cholesterol because it helps remove LDL (bad) cholesterol from your body-it helps keep the arteries clear.

One way to lower LDL cholesterol is to reduce your intake of trans fats; when you lower LDL cholesterol, HDL cholesterol increases-

What are some trans fats? Trans fats are invented as scientists began to "hydrogenate" liquid oils so that they can withstand better in food production and last longer. Trans fats are found in many commercially packaged foods, such as fried foods like French fries, some frying oils, packaged snacks, and hard stick butter...ect.

Avoid using cooking oils that are high in saturated fats/ trans fats such as coconut oil, palm oil or vegetable shortening.

To lower bad cholesterol, use vegetable oil, margarine, or fat free margarine instead of butter or shortening when cooking, or baking; use egg whites without the yellow yoke, or use egg substitute, eat more vegetables and grains, and lower your meat portions; eat very lean meats, and use fat free dairy products.

Another food product that we should try our very best to lessen our intake of is sugar.

The reason why we should try to lessen our sugar intake and manage it is because most of the foods that we eat contain a certain about of sugar-some more that others.

Our bodies take that sugar and turn it into glucose, sugar in the blood. The body uses glucose as its source of energy, but too much glucose in the blood over works the pancreas which supplies insulin to break down the glucose so the cells can use it; but if you eat too much sugar, you will have too much glucose in your blood, then the pancreas cannot make enough insulin to break it down. Too much glucose floating in your blood is called diabetes, which can be lethal to the body over a period of time-thus, is the reason why we should lessen our sugar intake, and because most of our foods have sugar, we must be watchful.

Some ways to decrease sugar intake:

- Instead of eating or cooking with regular sugar, use zero calorie sweeteners such as brands like SweetNLow, Natural Truvia, Splenda, Equal, NutraSweet, and SugarTwin; these will help reduce the glucose in your blood, thereby, lessening the work for your pancreas.
- Use fresh fruit, or fruit canned in water (not heavy syrup) to cook with.
- Decrease the amount of sugar in recipes.

- Stop drinking regular sodas, and substitute them with sugar free pops (if you just got to have a pop).
- Stay clear of most potato products, for most are full of sugar, some have more sugar than a regular candy bar.
- Remember, if its color is white, it is usually full of sugar, such as pasta, white bread, white flour, and white rice.

Read the content label on the foods that you buy; look for how many grams of sugar is in it, and don' forget to look at how many grams of carbohydrates it has-carbohydrates are just another form of sugar.

Remember, your body can get most of the sugar/ glucose that it needs just from the foods that we eat; you don't have to add those high sugar filled foods. It can be detrimental to good health.

I would be remiss if I didn't warn you to reduce your salt intake. While salt is a very necessary nutrient, too much of it can be harmful to your health

Table salt, or sodium chloride, its official name, gives electrolyte sodium to your diet. This mineral is essential for maintaining fluid balance within your cells. It also helps contracting your muscles and transmitting nerve impulses.

Salt also plays an important role in helping your digestive system absorb nutrients. You need about three grams of salt each day to maintain a healthy balance.

Too much salt has adverse side effects, such as:

- **Heart disease:** Almost 600,000 people die of heart disease in the United States every year; about one out of every four. Heart disease is the leading cause of death for both men and women, and more than half the deaths do to heart disease were men.
- **Water retention**: The amount of salt filled fluid on the outside of your cells determines the amount of water your body retains. If your salt intake is high, your kidneys cut back on the amount of water it releases into your urine so you can balance out the excess salt surrounding your cells. Thus, results in an increase blood volume due to water retention, which produces swelling in different parts of the body.
- **Dehydration**: dehydration defined is your body pulling water from within your cells. This is sometimes caused by too much salt intake. The

salt absorbs the water and causes your body to seek it from other parts of itself, which dehydrates you. Some symptoms of dehydration are: extreme thirst, nausea, dizziness, stomach cramps, vomiting and diarrhea. This is your body warning you of excess salt and trying to get rid of it by itself.

- **High blood pressure**: The higher the salt levels in your blood, the higher your blood volume, because your kidneys excrete less water in order to dilute the salt in your blood. Increases in salt, increased blood volume, which increases blood pressure because your body is constantly trying to maintain water balance among the cells.

While we are discussing the essential things that we should be sure to take into our bodies, I cannot stress enough of how important it is for you to take in enough water; this fact can never be overstated. Our bodies can go without a lot of things for a good long while, but water is so important to the proper functioning of our bodies until one can only go about three days without water-after which death soon occurs.

Water is very necessary to all living things-plants, animals, flowers etc. There is more water upon the earth than anything else. The earth is about 70% water, and because God created man from the earth, man water consistency is about the same. He is about 65% water.

70% water adds up to about 326 million trillion gallons resting in our oceans, lakes, rivers, and the clouds in the sky.

Water is all around us; it is in a constant cycle. It evaporates from the earth into the clouds, and then the clouds empty the water back to the earth; this cycle continues over and over again. It is how God supplies man with the water that he needs on a daily basis.

It has been said that we should consume about two to three liters of water a day; which includes all of our diet-the foods that we eat.

While it has been stated that we should consume about 64 ounces of water every day, however, to know the proper amount of water that each individual should consume a day, research says that you take your weight and divide it by 2, and that shall give you how many ounces of water you should consume each day; example, if you weigh 100 pounds, then you should take in about 50 ounces of water each day (14 ounces less than what has been generally recommended)-that does not include the water that is in your food supply.

You should be just as mindful of how much water you drink, as to how much you are not drinking, because drinking too much water can be harmful to you as well.

Simply put, I suggest that you listen to your body. It is the mechanism that God set up to measure your need for water. Different things determine your need for water; it varies, such as hot days, exercising, sweating, etc. When you are thirsty, just give your body some water.

One of the signs that you are drinking too much water is your urine is clear. Normal urine has a yellow tint; it is the kidneys getting rid of the impurities in your system.

Your kidneys process about 30 ounces of water an hour. Any more than that puts extra stress on the kidneys.

So, make sure you get your daily water intake, but make sure that you don't overdo it, and suffer from water intoxication.

God intended for us to live a long healthy life. It is His plan for us, but we can choose to deviate from His plan by living wrong and eating wrong.

When we don't watch what we eat, how much we eat, and how often we eat, then, we choose to live a short unhealthy life riddled by high blood pressure, diabetes, strokes, heart disease and the like.

I don't believe that it is impossible for us to live to be several hundred years old. We can eat to live, or eat to die.

PRAY THIS PRAYER FOR STRENGTH

Dear God, the Father of all the universe; the one that created me, I thank you for life health and strength, and all that you are yet doing in my life. I pray Father that you would give me the fortitude to eat those things that generate life and good health for me; lead me to the right foods, and give me the wisdom to choose a healthy style of life. I choose, this day, to live long, healthy, and prosperously….In Jesus name I pray….. Amen….Amen…..and Amen

Chapter Thirteen

A HOLY DECREE-
DECREE IT SO

So often, we forget that we are more than simply mere mortals; we are sons of God that are able to speak and declare the things that we desire by the power of God- and expect them to come to pass, and they shall be as we declared them.

We are supposed to have abundant life (much joy). Note what Jesus says in John 10:10:

> 10. The thief comes not, but for to steal, and to kill, and to destroy: I am come that they might have life, and that they might have it more abundantly.

He says that the enemy will come to destroy you, but He will not allow it. Jesus has promised us abundant life, so we should expect what Jesus promised-Abundant life.

Because of His son-ship, we can walk in our son-ship, which in essence, is again Jesus' son-ship. Observe what he says in John 16: 23-26:

> 23: And in that day you shall ask me nothing. Verily, verily, I say unto you, Whatsoever you shall ask the Father in my name, he will give it you.

24. Heretofore have you asked nothing in my name: ask, and you shall receive, that your joy may be full.

25. These things have I spoken unto you in proverbs: but the time comes, when I shall no more speak unto you in proverbs, but I shall show you plainly of the Father.

26. At that day you shall ask in my name: and I say not unto you, that I will pray the Father for you.

Jesus said that after he is risen and goes back to the Father, we can ask God anything, and He will do it for us. In other word, He restores our relationship back with the Father; so that like Jesus, whatever we ask, or decree, shall come to pass because we are no longer servants, but sons of God.

We must decree what will be in our lives; a decree is much more than just a mere declare. A decree is an official order, as of a government or a court.

In other words, you have the official power of God to decree prosperity in your life; to decree good health; to decree long life.

Decree a change in your life right now; decree it and walk in that for which you have decreed.

When you decree it, you must believe that whatsoever you have decreed will come to pass. You must arise and walk in what you expect God to do.

If you are asking for good health, you must start a good healthy diet with some degree of exercise, and expect good health to come forth, even if heretofore you have had bad health. Your decree will turn it around. What you do has to line up with what you say. If you are decreeing good health, but you are continuing to eat wrong, and exercise of any degree is non existence, then your "life style" will cancel out your decree.

Observe what the bible says about the importance of your faith having works with it. James 2: 14-20:

> 14. What does it profit, my brothers, though a man say he has faith, and have not works? Can faith save him?

> 15. If a brother or sister be naked, and destitute of daily food,

> 16. And one of you say unto them, Depart in peace, be you warmed and filled;

notwithstanding, you give them not those things which are needful to the body; what does it profit?

17. Even so faith, if it has not works, is dead, being alone.

18. Yes, a man may say, you have faith, and I have works: show me your faith without your works, and I will show you my faith by my works.

19. You believe that there is one God; you do well: the devils also believe, and tremble.

20. But will you know, O vain man, that faith without works is dead?

If you are decreeing financial blessings, then you must rise up and manage your money, and start sowing seeds in other people's lives, and sow some seeds in other venues so that God can pour back into your life.

Because we are children of God, whatsoever we say has merit. Angels and demons are always listening to what you say; that's why as a Believer, we must watch carefully of what we say. The angels are ready to assist you in performing the work that you have decreed, but the demons are listening and ready to use your very words against you.

Whatever you say, heaven agrees with you, and bring it to pass, thus, your words can be used against you. Note what the bible says of this matter in Matthew 18: 18:

18. Verily I say unto you, Whatsoever you shall bind on earth shall be bound in heaven: and whatsoever you shall loose on earth shall be loosed in heaven.

The Kingdom of heaven agrees with you; that is why your words can bind you are set you free.

If you decree it, you must walk, or live within the confines of what you have decreed.

Remember, decree it, expect it, and watch God work it out for you.

YOU HAVE NOT BECAUSE
YOU ASK NOT FOR IT
YOU ASKED FOR IT AND
DIDN'T RECEIVE IT
BECAUSE YOU WANTED IT
AMIDST YOUR GREED

James 4: 2-3

YOUR DECREE

I decree that I am healthy and attracting wealth. I am no longer where I used to be mentally or physically. I am a new creation. I decree new and better friends and associates in my life.

I decree that no weapon formed against me shall prosper. It shall be destroyed; those that rise up against me shall be defeated.

I decree that all the confusion and disabling trouble in my life be gone right now. I will turn around from my old ways of living that brought me death and old age.

I decree that I am getting my health back; my state of health is turning around for the better; be gone sickness, be gone disease, be gone debt, and be gone sorrow.

I decree that I shall have better days ahead of me than I have lived behind me. I shall have the means to help others aspire to their full potential.

I decree that doors of prosperity shall open for me so that I can sow into others life.

I decree that good people shall come into my life that shall help me become the best that I can be, and assist me in walking in my destiny; and those people that are not good for me, and mean me no good, shall flee from me. God shall open my eyes that I might see that they are not good for me, and shall strengthen my heart to be able to walk away from them, and be strong enough to allow them to walk out of my life.

I decree that whatever sickness or disease that have been plaguing me and attacking my body is now gone, or yet leaving.

I decree all of this by the power that Jehovah gave Adam, the first man before sin. I shall walk in the fullness of my destiny, and be an example of the power of God resting on human flesh.

I decree it so right now as a child of the most high God-Amen.

A CLOSING PRAYER

Father God Jehovah, I pray that you will bless abundantly the readers of this book; give them the needed strength to change their way of living, eating, and thinking.

Open our eyes deer Lord that we might see the blessings that you have placed before us, and give us the will and the fortitude to move forward, and to glean from the things that we have gone through.

Dear Lord let us be an example to others of how to eat and live so to have a long and prosperous life riddled with good health and strength.

Bless now Father; bless right now!!

We proclaim that this partition is already done by the power of Jehovah, in the name of Jesus.

Amen

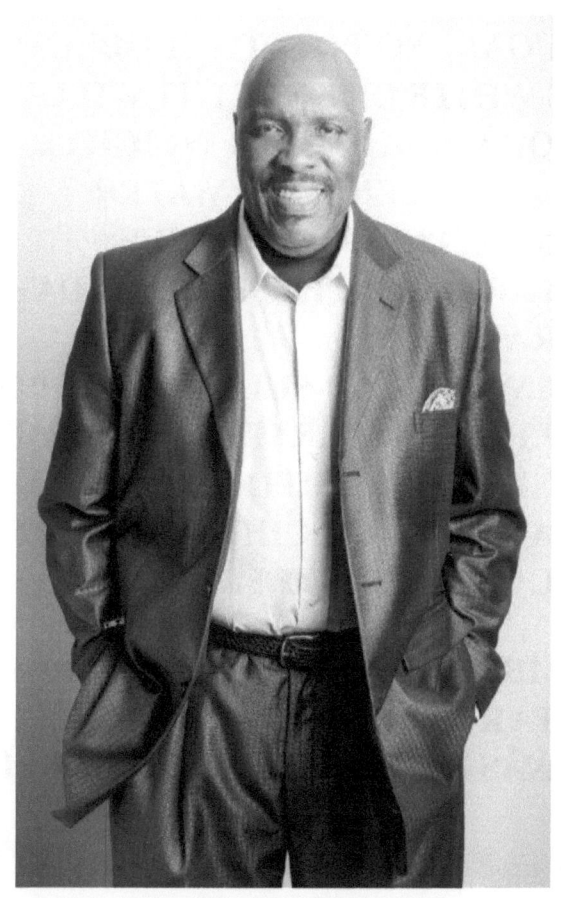

Picture after weight lost-220 pounds

LOSE 10 POUNDS IN TEN DAYS

1. **CUT OUT ALL CARBOHYDRATES FROM YOUR DIET!!!**
2. **NO BREAD, NO RICE, NO CANDY, NO SUGAR, NO POTATO PRODUCTS (IF IT IS WHITE OR SWEET, IT WILL DEFEAT YOU FROM LOSING WEIGHT).**
3. **DRINK PLENTY OF WATER**
4. **EXERCISE MODERATELY**
5. **START AND FINISH YOUR DAY WITH PRAYER**
6. **ALWAYS CONSULT YOUR DOCTOR BEFORE STARTING A DIET AND EXERCISE ROUTINE!!!!**
7. **EAT AS MUCH CHICKEN AND FISH AS YOU WANT (NOT FRIED).**

REMEMBER, STAY AWAY FROM BEEF AND PORK-PARTICULARLY PORK..........YOUR BODY WAS NEVER MEANT TO EAT MEAT!!

DRINK PLENTY OF WATER; A GREAT MANY

ILLNESSES BEGIN BECAUSE YOUR BODY DOES NOT HAVE ENOUGH WATER. YOU ARE OFTEN DEHYDRATED AND DON'T REALIZE IT.

STOP STRESSING AND WORRYING ABOUT THINGS THAT YOU CANNOT CHANGE; IF LEFT ALONE, MOST THINGS WILL FIX THEMSELVES; WORRYING ONLY PUTS MORE STRESS ON YOUR BODY, WHICH LEADS TO SICKNESS AND AN EARLY DEATH.

EAT A BALANCED DIET! THE OLDER YOU GET, THE MORE IMPORTANT A BALANCED DIET IS. AS YOU GET OLDER, YOU NEED TO ADD SOME VITAMINS IN YOUR DAILY DIET, SUCH AS ONE A DAY VITAMINS FOR MEN AND WOMEN, AND OTHER VITAMINS THAT IS SPECIFICLY FOR MEN AND WOMEN OVER 50.

VITAMINS HELP SUPPLIMENT WHAT YOU FAIL TO GET IN YOUR FOODS.

CONSISTANTLY FILL YOUR DAILY DIET WITH FOODS THAT ARE NATURAL ANTIOXIDANTS, AND FOODS THAT NATURALLY FIGHT INFLAMATION, SUCH AS BLUEBERRYS, BLACKBERRIES, RASBERRIES, KALE, DEEP GREEN LEAF VEGETABLES, ORANGES, APPLES, CANTALOPES, PRUNES, FIGS. IF YOU EAT SUCH THINGS AS THESE, AND STAY

AWAY FROM THOSE HARMFUL FOODS,
YOU WON'T HAVE TO GO TO THE DRUG
STORE TO PURCHASE SOME MEDICINE
TO CLEAN YOU OUT; THESE FRUITS AND
VEGETABLES WILL DO IT NATURALLY;
THEY WAY THAT GOD INTENTED IT TO BE.

THE MORE MEDICINE THAT YOU TAKE,
THE MORE YOUR BODY WILL ADAPT
TO THE MEDICINE, AND STOP OR SLOW
DOWN DOING THE THINGS THAT IT
WAS DESIGNED TO DO NATURALLY.

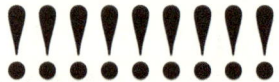

STOP EATING CERTAIN FOODS
AND SOME OF YOUR AILMENTS
WILL NATURALLY GO AWAY

SOMETIMES, WHAT YOU CALL SINUSES
IS MERELY YOUR BODY'S ALLERGIC
REACTION TO WHAT YOU ARE EATING.

WEIGHT YOURSELF ONCE A MONTH
SO THAT YOU WILL STAY IN TUNED
WITH WHERE YOU ARE IN YOUR WEIGHT

BELOVED, I WISH ABOVE ALL THINGS
THAT YOU MIGHT PROSPER AND BE IN
HEALTH, EVEN AS YOUR SOUL PROSPERS.

3 JOHN 1:2

NOTES

NOTES

NOTES

NOTES

NOTES

NOTES

NOTES

NOTES

NOTES

NOTES